Essential
Paediatric
Dermatology

For Hazel, my wife, who has sacrificed her leisure hours typing and retyping the manuscript, and for my children Daniel, Gina and Simon.

Essential Paediatric Dermatology

Julian Verbov, JP, MD, FRCP, FIBiol.

Consultant Paediatric Dermatologist,
Royal Liverpool Children's Hospital,
Liverpool, L7 7DG, UK.

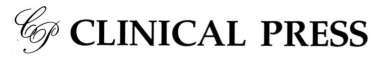 **CLINICAL PRESS**

Published by Clinical Press Limited.
Registered Office: The Coach House,
26 Oakfield Road, Clifton, Bristol, BS8 2AT

ISBN 1-85457-000-5

British Library Cataloguing in Publication Data

Verbov, Julian
    Essential paediatric dermatology.
    1. Pediatric dermatology
    I. Title
    618.92′5   RJ511

    ISBN 1-85457-000-5

Library of Congress Cataloguing-in-Publication Data

Verbov, Julian.
    Essential paediatric dermatology.

    Includes bibliographies and index.
    1. Pediatric dermatology.   I. Title. [DNLM: 1. Skin
Diseases—in adolescence.   2. Skin Diseases—in infancy
& childhood.   WS 260 V479e]
RJ511.V48   1988   618.92′5   88-797
ISBN 1-85457-000-5

Printed by Presscraft, Hartlebury, Worcs., UK
Bound by John Sherratt & Son, Manchester, UK

Contents

Acknowledgement

I am very grateful to Mr S. Gill, Chief Photographer of the Royal Liverpool Hospital Department of Medical Illustration for providing and allowing reproduction of many of the photographs in the book. I should like to thank colleagues who have permitted me to use photographs of their patients.

Preface

This is a concise textbook of paediatric dermatology. I have chosen the contents to include both common and uncommon disorders about which I believe some knowledge is essential. Generous use of colour illustrations serves to further aid diagnosis.

The aim is to provide a wider understanding of skin diseases in children both in their diagnosis and management with emphasis on everyday paediatric skin problems. I intend to concentrate on disorders regularly seen in my teaching clinics over many years and described in lectures to undergraduates, postgraduates and nurses.

It is of course important for any doctor to distinguish a sick child from a healthy one, not to miss the diagnosis of a serious condition and to know what and when to refer to a Consultant. However, if I were asked for practical purposes what were the skin disorders it was most essential to know about it would be the following: atopic dermatitis, impetigo, scabies, warts, papular urticaria, irritant napkin dermatitis, infantile seborrhoeic dermatitis and psoriasis.

Many diseases mentioned also occur in adults but their natural history and management is often different in children. I recognize the paediatric divisions—newborn (birth to one month), infancy (one month to two years), childhood (two to 12 years), and adolescence (12 to 16 years) but because so many conditions do occur at any age, I considered it more sensible not to divide the book artificially. However, a chapter on The Newborn was required but even here some of the conditions mentioned can occur at other ages or continue into infancy or childhood, and some conditions only mentioned elsewhere, e.g. Letterer–Siwe disease, may present in the newborn. Also some congenital conditions, e.g. sebaceous naevus, do not appear in The Newborn chapter because they are usually first noticed later on. I have tried to reduce overlap to a minimum although a few disorders do merit multiple mention.

I hope that a wide readership will include dermatologists in training, paediatricians, family practitioners, clinical medical officers, senior medical students and nurses.

It will be a source of satisfaction to me if this book stimulates further interest in this important and special branch of dermatology.

Julian Verbov
Royal Liverpool Children's Hospital,
Myrtle Street,
Liverpool

1

The Approach to Child and Parent

History-taking, examination and discussion of treatment should take place in a friendly, good-humoured atmosphere in a pleasantly decorated room with adequate lighting and heating. Both child and parents should feel at ease. The approach to the child with skin disease is often dictated by the parents' attitude to a visit to the doctor. Most parents treat the visit as part of everyday routine and will usually bring a child who is happy and cooperative. However, one also sees both immature parents unable to cope and irresponsible parents who refuse to cope. Of course one expects the young child to be shy at meeting a stranger (or strangers) but an intelligent parent will help the consultation to be a pleasant one. There are toys and picture books in my hospital consulting room and patients play with these while I talk in the same room to their parents about the relevant history of the complaint. I am quite happy for siblings to come into the consulting room at the same time.

When an eruption is widespread, my nurse organizes that the child undresses to underclothes before coming in to the clinic but if the child is loathe to undress he can do so when I see him. The child is usually examined on the couch but when necessary I examine an infant with a parent holding him.

It is important to remember that one is often treating or managing the parent rather than the child. Examining the spoilt child may present a problem but I explain to the parent how important it is for me to examine the whole skin. Spoiling a child is abusing it, although this is not as readily appreciated as neglect.

Many trivial or self-limiting complaints do not require a Consultant opinion but parents have often insisted on one and the family doctor has complied. At my children's hospital situated in a deprived area,

1

many children are referred to me via the Accident and Emergency Department and often the child has appeared there because the parents say they lack confidence in their family doctor, or his treatment has made the child worse, or they have not bothered to attend the doctor, or their own doctor has an appointment system and they can't wait to see him, etc. It is a modern-day phenomenon that many children I see are from one-parent families and may attend unaccompanied and others may be accompanied by a grandparent, sibling, family friend or social worker rather than by a parent. Occasionally, one finds parents who encourage their child's admission to hospital but then neither visit nor enquire of the child; a child in hospital needs parental love and attention.

Parents may just seek reassurance and thus it is most important to spend time explaining any particular worries they have. I emphasize to them how important it is not to allow their child to see that they are worried.

I prefer to explain treatment rather than to hand out written instructions regarding scabies or plantar warts, for instance; if such treatment is explained to parents, this is a more personal approach. More realistically, some adults are unable to read or understand written instructions so that verbal explanations are beneficial from this point of view. Use of topical steroid preparations is a common worry of parents, often derived from newspaper or other media publicity or from friends, and I emphasize that sparing and infrequent use is safe. I mention how topical steroids have revolutionized eczema management and how doctors try to prescribe mildly potent ones if there is a necessity for prolonged use. A parent innocently abusing a child with atopic dermatitis by feeding him an unproven and incomplete diet for unproven food intolerance can do more damage than topical steroids. Skin biopsy or removal of a lesion is occasionally necessary in paediatric practice and this should be performed under local (rather than general) anaesthetic if possible, and I usually prescribe a single dose of trimeprazine syrup pre-operatively in the younger child. A local anaesthetic cream has recently appeared producing good local anaesthesia; slow action is a disadvantage[1].

REFERENCE

1. Rutter, N. (1987). Drug absorption through the skin: a mixed blessing. *Arch. Dis. Child.*, **62**, 220–1.

2

The Newborn

CONTENTS

Epidermolytic hyperkeratosis (bullous ichthyosiform erythroderma)
Non-bullous ichthyosiform erythroderma
Lamellar ichthyosis
Collodion baby
X-linked (recessive) ichthyosis
Incontinentia pigmenti (Bloch–Sulzberger syndrome)
Epidermolysis bullosa (mechano-bullous diseases)
Simple epidermolysis bullosa
Junctional epidermolysis bullosa
Dystrophic epidermolysis bullosa
Autosomal recessive form
Autosomal dominant form
Neonatal lupus erythematosus

CUTIS MARMORATA

This is a normal reticulated bluish mottling of the skin seen on the trunk and extremities (Figure 2.1). It is a physiological response to chilling with resultant dilatation of capillaries and small venules and (unlike livedo reticularis, see Chapter 8) disappears with rewarming.

TOXIC ERYTHEMA OF THE NEWBORN

This common benign condition begins within 48 hours of birth and disappears in a few days. Blotchy erythematous macules 2–3 cm in diameter with a central vesicle, appear over trunk, face or limbs. A smear of the vesicle reveals numerous eosinophils.

TRANSIENT NEONATAL PUSTULOSIS *(Transient neonatal pustular melanosis)*

This is an uncommon benign self-limiting condition of unknown aetiology in which scanty superficial sterile pustules without associated erythema are present at birth (Figures 2.2 and 2.3). Neck and trunk are common sites, but lesions can occur anywhere. Individual pustules either disappear spontaneously within a few days, rupture and peel, or dry producing a flat brownish crust which can be gently scratched away[1]. New lesions may continue to appear for one or two weeks.

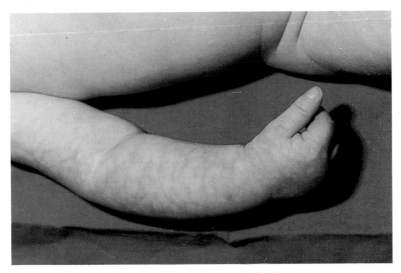

Figure 2.1 **Cutis marmorata** over thigh in a neonate.

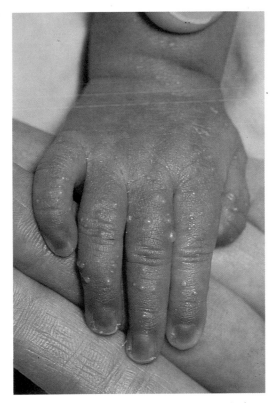

Figure 2.2 **Transient neonatal pustulosis** in a
2-week-old baby.

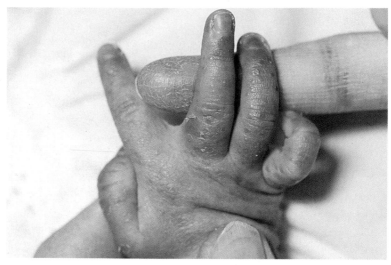

Figure 2.3   **Transient neonatal pustulosis**—finger lesions resolving at 18 days in same baby.

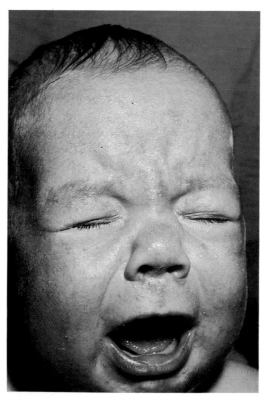

Figure 2.4   **Milia**. The small white papules can be seen over forehead, cheeks and inferior to nose.

MILIA

These lesions commonly occur on the face of the newborn and result from retention of keratin and sebaceous material within the pilosebaceous apparatus of the neonate (Figure 2.4). They appear as multiple pearly white or yellow 1–2 mm papules. These keratin cysts usually rupture onto the skin surface and disappear within a few weeks of birth.

SEBACEOUS GLAND HYPERPLASIA

This is manifested by multiple yellow tiny papules on the nose, cheeks and upper lips of newborn infants (Figure 2.5). They are a manifestation of maternal androgen stimulation and are a temporary phenomenon resolving in a few weeks. Although sometimes considered the same as milia, the sebaceous hyperplasia papules tend to be more florid and are not cystic.

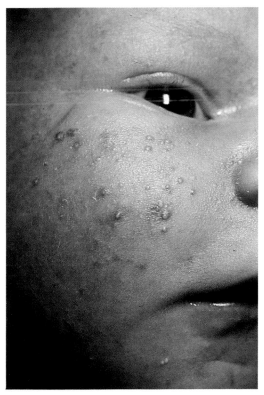

Figure 2.5   **Sebaceous gland hyperplasia** in a 23-day-old infant showing florid yellow papules.

MILIARIA

This is caused by eccrine sweat retention and is characterized by an erythematous papulo-vesicular eruption that is distributed particularly over the face, neck, upper chest and back but anywhere where there is excessive heating of the skin (Figure 2.6). Therapy is directed towards avoidance of excessive heat and humidity with lightweight loose clothing recommended.

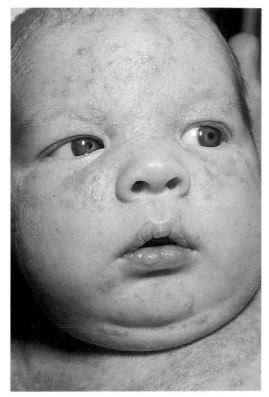

Figure 2.6 **Miliaria.** Face and chest lesions in a 3-week-old baby.

STAPHYLOCOCCAL INFECTIONS

Scalded skin syndrome

In this infection a widespread tender erythema develops within a few hours to a few days, worse over face, neck, axillae and groins. This is followed by the appearance of large flaccid bullae. The upper epidermis peels away leaving scald-like areas. Sometimes the eruption may be more localized (Figure 2.7) and erythema without blistering is

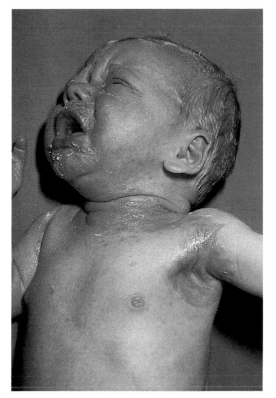

Figure 2.7 **Staphylococcal scalded skin syndrome.** Close-up of a 12-day-old child showing facial erythema and perioral, neck and axillary involvement.

also seen. A penicillinase-resistant penicillin or fusidic acid is indicated for this infection due to production of an exotoxin from phage Group 2 benzylpenicillin-resistant staphylococci. Recovery is within 5–7 days. There is often a history of typical impetigo in a sibling. (See also Chapter 4.)

Bullous impetigo

This is a purely bullous or vesicular form of impetigo seen particularly in the newborn (Figures 2.8 and 2.9). Lesions grow only staphylococci on culture. Treatment is as for staphylococcal scalded skin syndrome.

CONGENITAL LYMPHOEDEMA

Lymphoedema indicates diffuse soft-tissue swelling caused by accumulation of lymph as a result of inadequate lymphatic drainage.

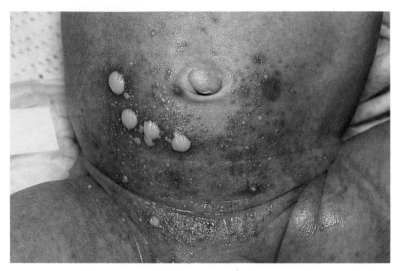

Figure 2.8   **Bullous impetigo** in a 12-day-old baby.

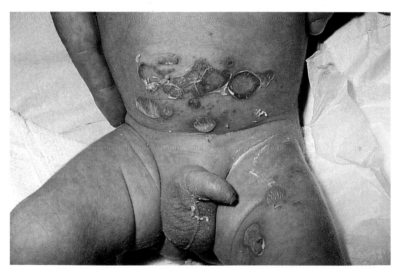

Figure 2.9   **Bullous impetigo.** Another baby, two weeks old, showing bullae, some of which clearly show a fluid level of pus. Began at 9 days.

In congenital lymphoedema the area involved is swollen at birth. The swelling is firm and pits on pressure. When occurring in females and if hypoplastic. toenails are present, *Turner's Syndrome* should be suspected.

DISORDERS OF SUBCUTANEOUS FAT

Neonatal cold injury

This is a benign self-limiting condition seen occasionally in healthy but often premature newborn babies in the first few weeks of life (Figure 2.10). Pitting oedema more marked over limbs may co-exist with a few sharply-defined woody indurated non-pitting areas of skin feeling cold to the touch. Buttocks and back are favoured areas for the hardened skin but such areas may occur anywhere. Management consists of ensuring that the child is kept adequately warm, and spontaneous resolution leaving no permanent skin change is to be expected within a week or so.

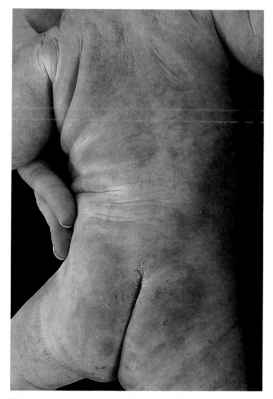

Figure 2.10 **Cold injury** in a 3-week-old baby. Baby was delivered by Caesarean section and skin change, particularly of buttocks which felt like cold wooden blocks, became visible at 18 days. Indurated skin in folds over back is also seen. No central heating at home.

It should be noted that the change in the subcutaneous fat giving rise to the hardened skin in neonatal cold injury is termed *sclerema* and in babies where sclerema is prominent, widespread and more prolonged, there may be no history of exposure to cold but there is often evidence of underlying preexisting disease which must be investigated.

Subcutaneous fat necrosis

This is a similar entity to neonatal cold injury seen particularly in healthy full-term or postmature neonates in the first six weeks of life. It is associated with firm nodules of various sizes not attached to deeper structures: there is no pitting oedema.

NAEVI

Pigmented naevi

Café-au-lait patches These hyperpigmented macules with well-defined borders are usually of no pathological significance (Figure 2.11). However, before puberty five or more patches greater than 0.5 cm in

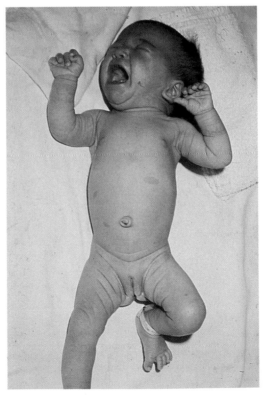

Figure 2.11   **Café-au-lait patches** (three are visible) over abdomen in a 6-week-old baby.

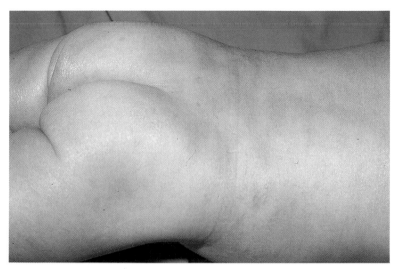

Figure 2.12 **Mongolian patches** in a Pakistani infant. Note the slate-grey appearance of lesions.

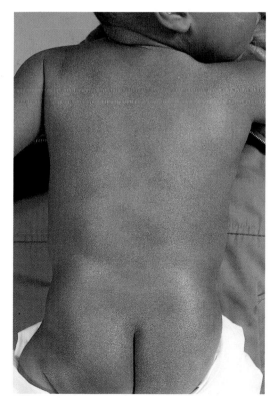

Figure 2.13 **Mongolian patches** in a Nigerian infant. Lesions have a blacker appearance in this darker-skinned child.

diameter are presumptive evidence of neurofibromatosis. (See also Neurofibromatosis, Chapter 10).

Mongolian patches   These congenital macular slate grey or black patches are generally found over lumbosacral areas and buttocks but they can occur anywhere on the skin including the face (Figures 2.12 and 2.13). Most negro and oriental babies show them but they are also present in less than 10% of caucasoids. They usually disappear by the end of the first decade. They represent collections of spindle-shaped melanocytes located deep in the dermis. It is important to distinguish them from bruises such as may be seen in non-accidental injury.

Giant pigmented naevus   This is a special form of melanocytic naevus which presents at birth as an extensive pigmented hairy area often occupying the lower abdomen and buttocks to cover the bathing-trunks' area (Figure 2.14). Such naevi occur less frequently

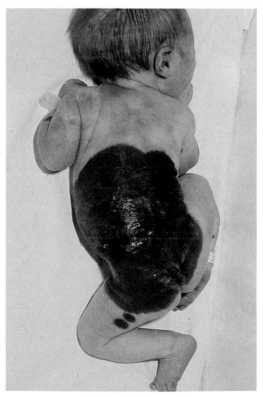

Figure 2.14   **Giant pigmented naevus** in a 2-day-old girl. The erosion visible and present at birth healed within a few days. The pigmentation has become paler over the last 7 years but many more pigmented naevi, often hairy, have appeared over the body. Some have been excised.

elsewhere. Treatment consists of early surgical excision wherever possible because of the risk of malignant change in lesions. The risk is in the region of 6% and malignant change most commonly occurs during the first decade. There has been a useful written symposium recently on the management of congenital naevocytic naevi[2].

Vascular Naevi

Salmon patch   This is a common congenital macular pink area with distended capillaries situated over the forehead, glabella, upper eyelids and nape of neck (Figure 2.15). No treatment is necessary because lesions fade in the first year of life with the exception of the nuchal lesion (so-called 'stork bite') which tends to persist but usually becomes covered by hair and is thus unnoticed.

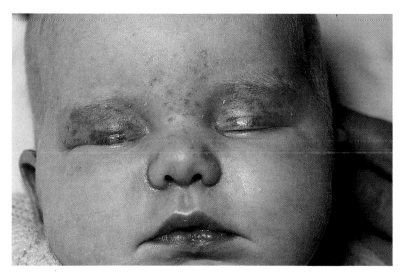

Figure 2.15   **Salmon patches.** Striking lesions over eyelids.

Port-wine stain *(naevus flammeus)*   This is always present at birth and is composed of irregularly dilated endothelial-lined capillary vessels confined to the upper dermis; no proliferation of endothelial cells is seen (Figure 2.16). They do not involute although some fade in colour slightly. They may, in fact, grow additional dilated vessels, particularly over the face, and these can bleed. Port-wine stains may occur at any skin site and there may be adjacent mucosal involvement. However, they are seen most commonly over head and neck. Those involving the supraorbital region are particularly likely to be associated with similar lesions involving the meninges on the same

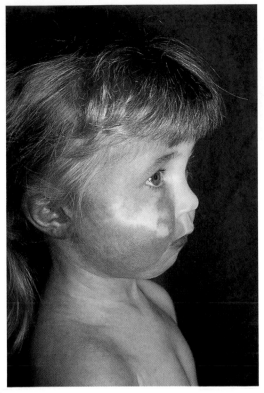

Figure 2.16   **Port-wine stain.** This extensive lesion in a 2½-year-old child was visible at birth.

side, constituting the *Sturge–Weber syndrome*. Manifestations of Sturge–Weber syndrome such as epilepsy and hemiplegia may appear in the first year of life but would be unusual to present in the neonate. An association of facial port-wine stain with congenital glaucoma should be appreciated, particularly as the glaucoma is usually asymptomatic early in life. Cosmetic cover remains the recommended treatment of port-wine stains but further development in laser therapy may make this a useful tool in some older children in the future.

Strawberry mark *(capillary haemangioma)* This is not usually present at birth but generally appears in the first month of life (Figures 2.17 and 2.18). Prematurity appears to be a predisposing factor in the appearance of these capillary lesions[3]. Common sites are head, neck and trunk. They appear as well-defined small telangiectatic areas and grow to raised red lobulated tumours with capillaries visible over the surface. They grow rapidly with the child in the first year of life and

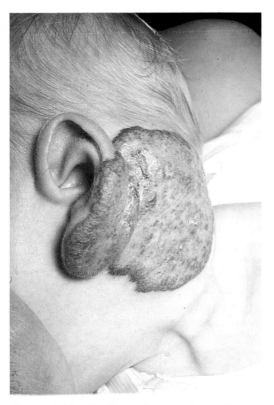

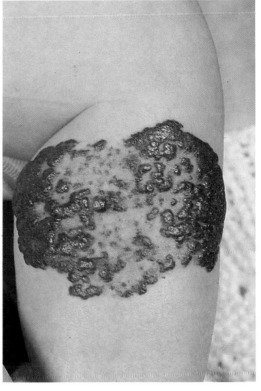

Figure 2.17 **Capillary haemangioma (straw-berry mark).** Large haemangioma both behind and affecting the pinna.

Figure 2.18 **Capillary haemangioma (straw-berry mark).** This large lesion over the leg in this 12-week-old girl had appeared within the first month of life. At follow-up 14 months later, it was all resolving nicely. The author often shows parents a standard series of photos illustrating the natural resolution of even large lesions.

then become stationary, involuting usually completely, over the next 4–5 years. Residual scarring may follow the occasional, often fric-tional lesion, that bleeds slightly, becomes infected, or ulcerates. Haemangiomas that grow rapidly or appear at vital structures such as the eyes, larynx, or pharynx may merit treatment with short-term systemic corticosteroid therapy to encourage involution.

Cavernous haemangioma This can really be considered to be the same as a strawberry mark, only deeper. Lesions are composed of larger mature vascular elements with involvement of both dermis and subcutaneous tissue. They are seen as bluish-red areas with indistinct borders. They do not grow as rapidly as strawberry marks. It is not

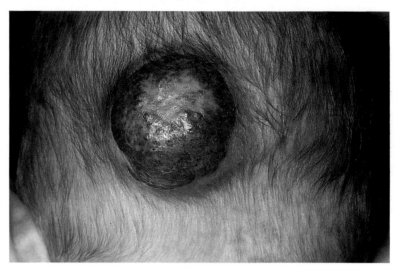

Figure 2.19 **Mixed haemangioma.** This 5-month-old infant has a capillary haemangioma with a minor subcutaneous element.

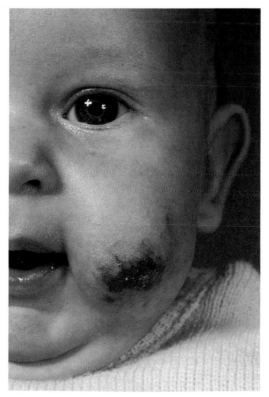

Figure 2.20 **Mixed haemangioma.** There is a marked subcutaneous element in this lesion in this 3 month-old child.

uncommon for *mixed forms* of strawberry and cavernous haemangioma to occur (Figures 2.19 and 2.20). These lesions also resolve but resolution may be incomplete.

The rare *Kasabach–Merritt syndrome*, in which there is thrombocytopenia caused by platelet sequestration and destruction, occurs especially but not only in giant cavernous haemangiomas. Such infants would of course be admitted to hospital and treatment would include whole blood or platelet transfusions and short-term systemic corticosteroids.

GENODERMATOSES

Ichthyoses

Harlequin foetus   This clinical syndrome is the most severe form of ichthyosis. The foetus is born prematurely and is of low birth weight. The baby is covered with thick armour-like skin which is split by deep fissures into polygonal plates. Respiratory movements are restricted and death usually occurs in the first few weeks of life because of this and restriction of feeding. The pattern of inheritance is autosomal recessive[4]. A successfully treated baby with this condition has recently been described and mention is made of the importance of fluid balance[5].

Epidermolytic hyperkeratosis *(bullous ichthyosiform erythroderma)*
In this autosomal dominant condition (Figures 2.21 and 2.22) areas of epidermis peel away shortly after birth leaving raw areas and the appearance may suggest epidermolysis bullosa (see later). The next stage is of crops of bullae which burst to leave raw areas that heal rapidly, but have a tendency to become secondarily infected. The background skin is erythematous. In time, warty hyperkeratosis becomes more prominent, appearing strikingly linear in the flexures. Histopathology reveals hydropic degeneration of the Malpighian cells. As the cells migrate up from the basal layer there is nuclear shrinkage and increasing vacuolation of the cytoplasm. Careful handling of the skin, emollients, antiseptic dressings and antibiotic therapy when necessary, will be required. The condition can be diagnosed prenatally by foetoscopy and foetal skin biopsy[6].

Non-bullous ichthyosiform erythroderma   This is an autosomal recessive disorder (Figures 2.23 and 2.24) which may present as a 'collodion baby' (see below) in which case the true nature will become

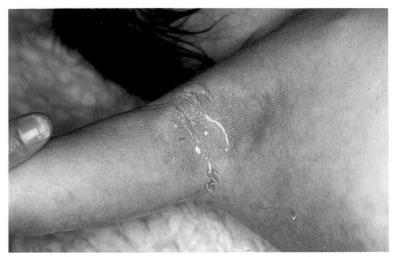

Figure 2.21   **Epidermolytic hyperkeratosis.** This 3-month-old boy showed widespread superficial readily healing blisters as a neonate. The slide shows a rather raw right axilla.

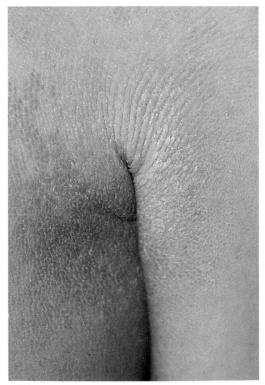

Figure 2.22   **Epidermolytic hyperkeratosis.** The same child as in Figure 2.21 at 4½ years showing chronic linear corrugated hyperkeratotic skin over left anterior axillary fold.

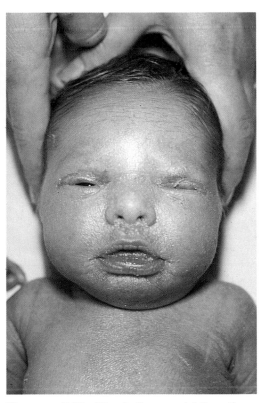

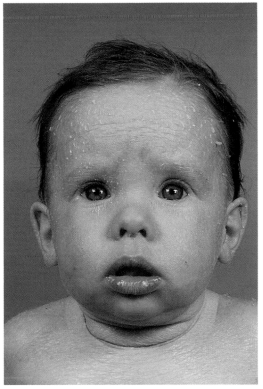

Figure 2.23 **Non-bullous ichthyosiform erythroderma** in a 4-day-old female collodion baby.

Figure 2.24 **Non-bullous ichthyosiform erythroderma.** Same girl as in Figure 2.23 at 9 months showing fine white scaling and faintly red skin.

apparent after the membrane peels off. However, it can also present as such at birth, with the entire skin dull red but more marked in the flexures. Superimposed on the erythema are fine white scales. There may be ectropion. The severity of the condition varies but most patients survive and improve, showing generalized faint erythema, and hyperkeratosis, most marked over palms and soles, as time goes on.

Lamellar ichthyosis This can be considered a generally more severe, but less common, form of autosomal recessive ichthyosis than non-bullous ichthyosiform erythroderma (Figures 2.25–2.27). Large greyish-brown scales with raised edges occur. There is normal hydrocarbon (alkane) content in scales compared to a marked increase in non-bullous ichthyosiform erythroderma. Emollients are essential in the management of the skin, and usually this is the only therapy required. Oral synthetic retinoid therapy does have a place in severe

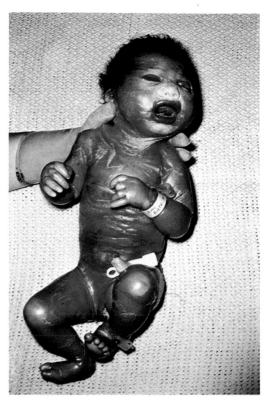

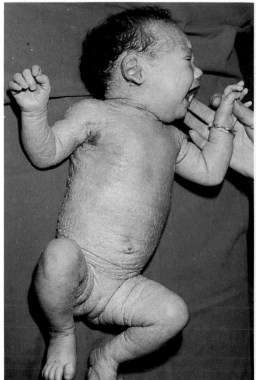

Figure 2.25 **Lamellar ichthyosis.** Collodion baby on first day of life.

Figure 2.26 **Lamellar ichthyosis.** Same child as in Figure 2.25 at 27 days showing how membrane has separated revealing dry skin.

debilitating disease, but apart from typical side effects, the risk of skeletal toxicity must be considered[7].

Collodion baby This describes an appearance rather than a specific disease (Figures 2.23 and 2.25). These babies are born enveloped in a shiny transparent but fairly rigid membrane which cracks and peels off after a few days, and at this time the true skin appearance of the child can be visualized. In fact, many of these children will have no underlying disorder but an appreciable number will have non-bullous ichthyosiform erythroderma, lamellar ichthyosis, X-linked ichthyosis, or ichthyosis vulgaris.

X-linked (recessive) ichthyosis This is less common but more severe than the later-appearing ichthyosis vulgaris. The scales tend to be much larger, polygonal and have a dirty brown or black colour (Figure 2.28). The scaliness is frequently obvious at birth. The entire skin

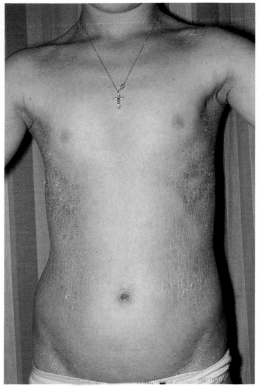

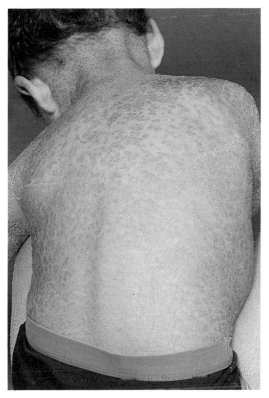

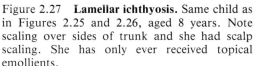

Figure 2.27 **Lamellar ichthyosis.** Same child as in Figures 2.25 and 2.26, aged 8 years. Note scaling over sides of trunk and she had scalp scaling. She has only ever received topical emollients.

Figure 2.28 **X-linked ichthyosis.** Boy of 2 years with dark scales over back and back of neck.

surface including flexures and scalp may be affected but if the face is involved it is usually only the sides, and increased palm and sole markings are not a feature. The condition is persistent. Steroid sulphatase deficiency is associated with this disorder and its absence permits identification of maternal carriers. Urea-containing emollient creams are helpful.

Incontinentia pigmenti *(Bloch–Sulzberger syndrome)*

This is an X-linked dominant ectodermal dysplasia which usually presents within a few days of birth generally being prenatally lethal in males, the few surviving males being the result of spontaneous mutation. Linear or grouped vesicles appear on the trunk and limbs (Figures 2.29 and 2.30) but by the end of the first month blistering

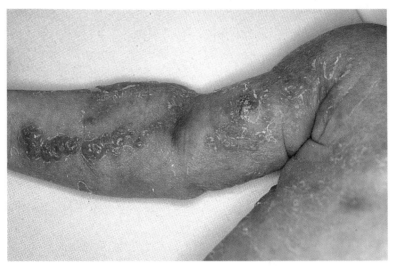

Figure 2.29 **Incontinentia pigmenti.** 11-day-old-female with linear blistering.

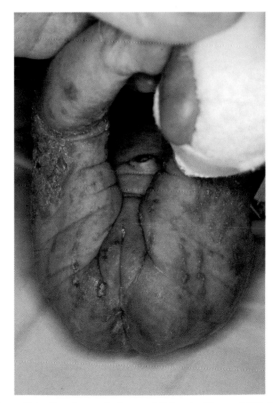

Figure 2.30 **Incontinentia pigmenti.** Same child as in Figure 2.29 showing blistering elsewhere in a typical striking distribution.

disappears and is usually followed by the appearance of small firm papules and warty plaques. The papules in turn involute leaving angulated and streaked pigmentation; hypopigmentation may also be visible. The condition is frequently associated with dental, skeletal, eye and central nervous system abnormalities which must be looked for.

Epidermolysis bullosa *(mechano-bullous diseases)*

Epidermolysis bullosa indicates a group of inherited non-inflammatory disorders in which blisters and erosions occur with mechanical, often minor, trauma. In the scarring, so-called *dystrophic forms*, pathology occurs beneath the basement membrane so that these scarring conditions *are sometimes referred to as dermolytic bullous dermatoses*. Prenatal diagnosis of mechano-bullous diseases by foetoscopy and skin biopsy has been performed on many occasions but the benefits and potential risks must always be carefully evaluated. There are many types of epidermolysis bullosa but mention shall only be made of some of the main ones.

Simple epidermolysis bullosa This is a widespread condition inherited as an autosomal dominant (Figure 2.31). The onset is usually within the first few months of life although erosions due to skin trauma at the time of birth can be present. Blisters which are formed by disintegration of basal and and suprabasal cells vary in size and rapidly become tense with clear fluid. The condition tends to be worse in warm weather. Mucous membranes are rarely affected. Secondary bacterial infection is common but healing without scarring follows. In this condition improvement often occurs with increasing age and protection of the skin from mechanical trauma is the mainstay of management.

Junctional epidermolysis bullosa In this severe autosomal recessive condition, which is frequently lethal in infancy, there is separation between the basement membrane and the basal cell plasma membrane and it is thus appropriately termed 'junctional'. There is severe skin and mucosal involvement, nails and teeth become dystrophic, and unlike simple epidermolysis bullosa, eroded areas heal slowly. Blisters may be haemorrhagic and are frequently secondarily infected. Genetic counselling is important. Patients who survive beyond the first 2–3 years of life develop many of the complications seen in severe recessive dermolytic bullous dermatosis[8].

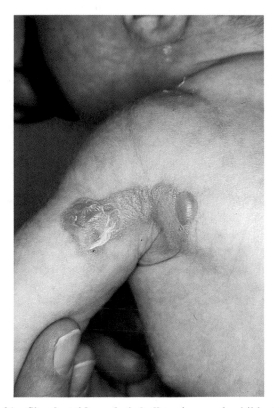

Figure 2.31   **Simple epidermolysis bullosa** in a male child at 19 days.

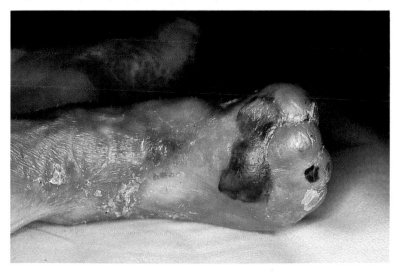

Figure 2.32   **Dystrophic epidermolysis bullosa**. Foot of female infant with recessive disease showing marked scarring. (Courtesy of Dr. M. Molokhia.)

Dystrophic epidermolysis bullosa *Autosomal recessive form* This severe scarring form usually appears at birth with minor trauma producing blistering and separation of epidermis. Mucous membranes are affected and mouth blisters and erosions which are sometimes haemorrhagic, are common. Pharyngeal and oesophageal involvement may produce strictures. Hands and feet are particularly affected and healing of these deeper blisters can produce syndactyly, requiring plastic surgery at a later date (Figure 2.32). Nails are dystrophic and milia in scarred areas are usual. This is a severe crippling form of disease and genetic counselling should be offered to parents of such children. Systemic steroid therapy can be of help to these patients but will affect growth and give rise to other toxic effects in the dosage required. More recently, phenytoin (diphenylhydantoin) a collagenase inhibitor, has been found to be effective in some patients with this disorder or junctional epidermolysis bullosa[9, 10], being prescribed because of evidence of increased levels of collagenase in both blistered and non-blistered areas of skin. However, it should be noted that phenytoin also has many side-effects.

Autosomal dominant form In this mild form which usually presents in early infancy or childhood, blisters heal leaving superficial discoloured scars particularly over hands, feet, elbows and knees. Nails may be dystrophic and milia are a common finding at the sites of healed blisters.

NEONATAL LUPUS ERYTHEMATOSUS

This is a rare condition in which neonates show discoid scaling erythematous lesions primarily over the face which resolve often leaving some atrophy. There is an associated increased incidence of systemic manifestations, especially congenital heart block. Both mother and child are usually positive for the anti-Ro/SSA antibody and generally show a speckled pattern of fluorescent antinuclear antibodies (ANA). The mother may not show any clinical evidence of systemic lupus erythematosus but may develop it later. Neonates with lupus erythematosus do have an increased risk of developing systemic lupus erythematosus when older[11] although lesions resolve and serological markers are usually lost within the first year. This is an important diagnosis to consider in the neonate presenting with a facial eruption. ESR, and other haematological and serological studies in mother and child are obviously necessary and the baby will require an ECG and perhaps a skin biopsy also. There is a useful recent review of neonatal lupus erythematosus[12].

Some other conditions that may present in the newborn are discussed later in more detail: infantile seborrhoeic dermatitis (Chapter 5); naevi (Chapter 7); Letterer–Siwe disease (Chapter 7); genodermatoses (Chapter 10).

REFERENCES

1. Merlob, P., Metzker, A. and Reisner, S. H. (1982). Transient neonatal pustular melanosis. *Am. J. Dis. Child.,* **136**, 521-2
2. Jacobs, A. H., Hurwitz, S., Prose, N. S., Rhodes, A. R., Alper, J. C., Bauer, B. S., Bader, K., Lucky, A. W., From, L., Spraker, M. K., Williams, M. L., Sagebiel, R. S., Vasconez, L. O., Norins, A. L., Treadwell, P. A. and Solomon, L. M. (1984). The management of congenital nevocytic nevi. *Pediatr. Dermatol.* **2**, 143-56
3. Amir, J., Metzker, A., Krikler, R. and Reisner, S. H. (1986). Strawberry haemangioma in preterm infants. *Pediatr. Dermatol.* **4**, 331-2
4. Unamuno, P., Pierola, J. M., Fernandez, E., Roman, C and Velasco, J. A. (1987). Harlequin foetus in four siblings. *Br. J. Dermatol.,* **116**, 569-72
5. Lawlor, F. and Peiris, S. (1985). Harlequin fetus successfully treated with etretinate. *Br. J. Dermatol.,* **112**, 585-90
6. Williams, M. L. (1983). The ichthyoses—pathogenesis and prenatal diagnosis: A review of recent advances. *Pediatr. Dermatol.,* **1**, 1-24
7. Tsambaos, D., Hilt, K. and Goos, M. (1987). Treatment of genodermatoses with oral retinoids: risk of bone changes. In Happle, R. and Grosshans, E. (eds.) *Pediatric Dermatology,* pp. 41-5. (Basle: Springer–Verlag)
8. Cooper, T. W. and Bauer, E. A. (1984). Epidermolysis bullosa: a review. *Pediatr. Dermatol.,* **1**, 181-8
9. Rogers, R. B., Yancey, K. B., Allen, B. S. and Guill, M. F. (1983). Phenytoin therapy for junctional epidermolysis bullosa. *Arch. Dermatol.,* **119**, 925-6
10. Armoni, M., Schlesinger, M., Vardy, P. A. and Metzker, A. (1985). Phenytoin and junctional epidermolysis bullosa. *Arch. Dermatol.,* **121**, 168 9
11. Lumpkin, III, L. R., Hall, J., Hogan, J. D., Tucker, S. B. and Jordon, R. E. (1985). Neonatal lupus erythematosus. A report of three cases associated with anti Ro/SSA antibodies. *Arch. Dermatol.,* **121**, 377-81
12. Korkij, W. and Soltani, K. (1984). Neonatal lupus erythematosus: a review. *Pediatr. Dermatol.,* **1**, 189-95

3

Atopic and Other Dermatitis

CONTENTS

ATOPIC DERMATITIS

The term 'atopy' indicates an inherited tendency to develop one or more of a related group of conditions (asthma, eczema of atopic type, allergic rhinitis, acute urticaria of allergic type) subject to much environmental influence. More than 10% of the British population are atopic, and allergic rhinitis is the most common manifestation.

Atopic eczema affects about 3% of children under the age of 5 years and produces much personal and family distress. The cause is unknown, and there is no convincing evidence yet that food intolerance, including food allergy, is more than occasionally present or relevant. Raised serum IgE concentrations are a secondary phenomenon found in 80% of atopics and one study of adults with atopic eczema concluded that a raised IgG4 concentration in atopic eczema is a monitor of prolonged exposure to an allergen that initiated an IgE response[1]. There is clearly, however, much more to atopic eczema than simply allergy.

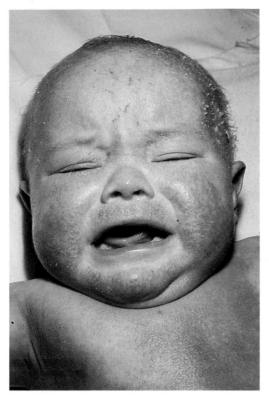

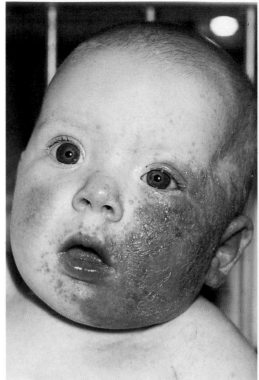

Figure 3.1 **Atopic dermatitis.** A 5-month-old male with excoriated eczema.

Figure 3.2 **Atopic dermatitis.** A 6-month-old female with mainly unilateral facial eczema. A day or so later the right side of her face flared also.

Clinical Features (Figures 3.1–3.13)

Mention of atopic eczema immediately brings to mind the baby vigorously rubbing his itchy head on the bedding and the older infant toddling along scratching or rubbing his itchy dry skin, making it painful and himself miserable. The ability to have a coordinated scratch does not occur before the age of 2 months. One also sees the older child, the adolescent, and even the adult, however, scratching more methodically and with exacerbations often related to stress at home, school, or work.

Although usually presenting between the ages of 3 months and 2 years, atopic eczema may first appear after the age of 2 years, and onset may sometimes be delayed until late childhood or adult life. Eczema beginning after the age of 2 years and prolonged extensor limb

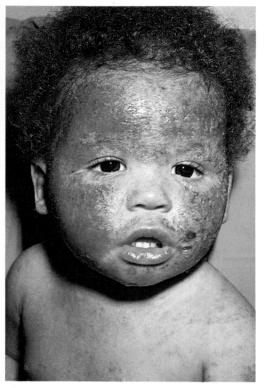

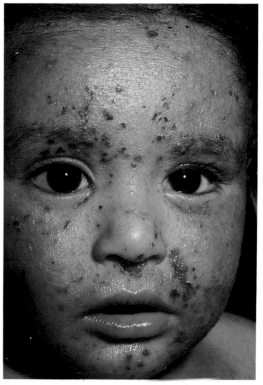

Figure 3.3 **Atopic dermatitis.** Severe excoriated eczema in a 15 month-old child.

Figure 3.4 **Atopic dermatitis.** Excoriated and infected eczema in a 11-month-old child.

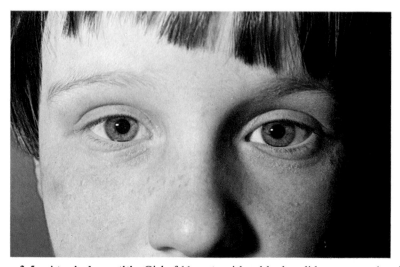

Figure 3.5 **Atopic dermatitis.** Girl of 11 years with rubbed eyelid eczema and typical extra infraorbital creases visible.

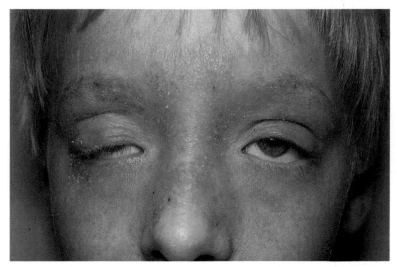

Figure 3.6 **Atopic dermatitis.** Infected eyelids following repeated rubbing in a boy of 9 years. This boy had been rubbing his eyelids for years and ophthalmological referral months before this photograph was taken had revealed eczematous reaction in both eyes particularly on the right where there was pannus formation in the cornea.

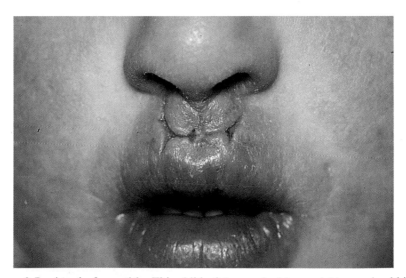

Figure 3.7 **Atopic dermatitis.** This child of 4 years had been picking and rubbing below the nose for months: the inflammation gradually resolved.

involvement both tend to have a poorer prognosis. Affected individuals have a one in four chance of developing asthma or allergic rhinitis, or both, sometime later.

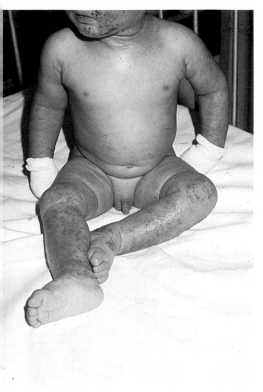

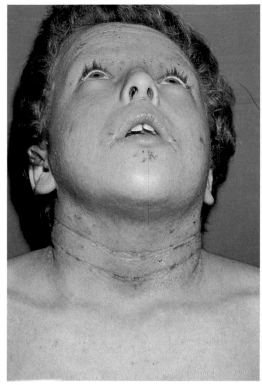

Figure 3.8 **Atopic dermatitis.** Extensor limb involvement in a boy of 11 months.

Figure 3.9 **Atopic dermatitis.** Lichenified eczema affecting the neck in a boy of 10 years—a common site.

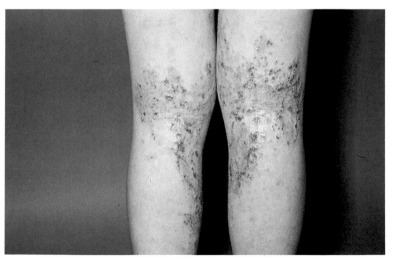

Figure 3.10 **Atopic dermatitis.** Excoriated infected eczema affecting popliteal fossae.

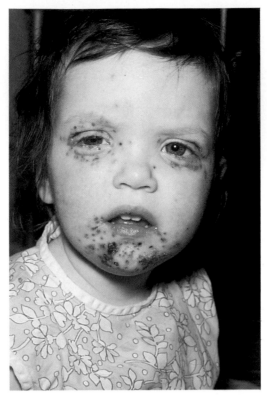

Figure 3.11 **Atopic dermatitis.** Eczema herpeticum over face. The discrete simplex lesions are secondarily infected.

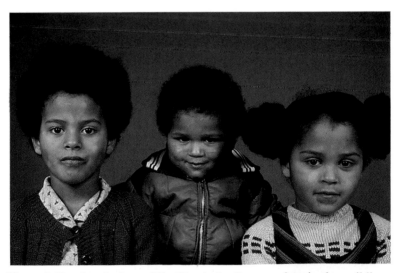

Figure 3.12 **Atopic dermatitis.** Pityriasis alba over face in three siblings.

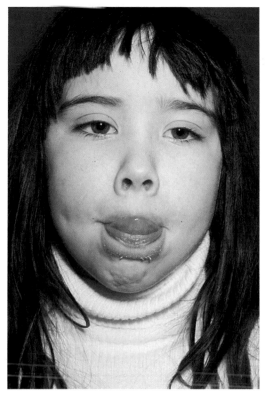

Figure 3.13 **Atopic dermatitis.** Lip-licking demonstrated. Most lip lickers are atopic.

Commonly affecting the face or scalp initially, eczema later affects the extensor aspect of the limbs and then localizes to the flexures, including cubital and popliteal fossae. Although buttocks may be affected in infants, there can be widespread skin involvement with sparing of the napkin area. Within months of onset cubital and popliteal fossae, lower buttock folds, and frictional areas such as neck, wrists and ankles become affected and eczema may sometimes be localized to these areas. When the front of the neck is involved the neck is often held stiffly. The dorsal aspect of hands, fingers and feet are other common sites. Patients with atopic eczema tend to have a *characteristic facial pallor*, may show *extra wrinkling below the eyelids* mainly as a result of rubbing and old oedema, and are often *lip lickers*. Eyelid eczema and dry cracked lips are common. Patchy skin roughness particularly over backs of upper arms and front of thighs due to horny plugging of follicles (keratosis pilaris) is common both in atopics and non-atopics. *Pityriasis alba,* in which scaling and hypopigmented patches appear particularly over facial skin is seen most commonly and more easily in dark-skinned individuals. Follicular papules are a prominent feature in the black child with atopic dermatitis. *Lichenification*, indicating a peculiar thickening of the skin due to persistent rubbing and scratching with accentuation of skin markings is a common finding. Sometimes hair may be lost in eczema areas due to the trauma of repeated rubbing. *Reticulate pigmentation* over front and sides of neck is sometimes seen[2]. Rubbing and scratching encourage secondary bacterial infection and painless lymphadenopathy is frequently found with inflamed skin. *White dermographism*, which is easily elicited over the back presents as white macular areas when light pressure is applied to the skin. It is due to capillary constriction and is often pronounced if eczema is active over the trunk.

The affected individual has dermatitis, and his skin is prone to secondary bacterial and viral infection and sweat retention. Viral warts are often more profuse probably as a result of defective cell-mediated immunity; unfortunately their spread is encouraged by use of the often necessary topical corticosteroids. The skin of children with atopic eczema is commonly dry, and some children inherit a tendency to both atopic dermatitis and autosomal dominant ichthyosis vulgaris. As in ichthyosis vulgaris, increased palmar and plantar markings may be present.

Investigations

If clinically, food intolerance seems to be a factor in the worsening of atopic eczema, a short-term elimination diet can be given (see later); a recent study in adults suggested that antigen absorption from the gut may play a role in the aetiopathogenesis of atopic eczema[3]. Prick testing to detect food allergy is unreliable in young children, and in patients with active eczema some positive results are often merely a reflection of the state of skin reactivity at the time of testing. Performing hyposensitization to ingested (or inhaled) allergens so shown will not improve atopic eczema and is not recommended. Sometimes more useful, particularly if it confirms a clinical impression, is a radio-allergosorbent test on blood, which will indicate the IgE concentration and the materials against which IgE is directed—for example, milk, egg, or house-dust mite. Many patients with clinically proven food intolerance have negative skin and blood tests, suggesting that not only IgE but other immunological or non-immunological mechanisms are responsible[4]. Thus IgG, immune complexes, or non-immunological mechanisms, including psychological, pharmacological, toxic reactions or enzyme defects, may be relevant.

Management

Many children with atopic eczema are managed perfectly well by their family doctor without ever requiring hospital referral, and there are those with mild eczema whose parents do not even consult their own family doctor. It is a measure of the problem however, that each year nearly 20% of the new child outpatient referrals that I see have atopic eczema.

At the first interview it is important both to enquire about, and to listen to, the history of the condition from the parent and to be seen to listen; factors important to that particular child may thus be revealed. Atopic eczema affects the individual but influences the whole family, and treatment must be directed both towards the parents and the child.

Wool next to the skin must be avoided and cotton clothing is recommended. Too frequent bathing will make dry skin drier, and when washing a soap substitute such as aqueous cream or emulsifying ointment can be used, and one of the many proprietary emollient preparations available can be added to bath water. Dry skin whether associated with atopy or not is prone to frictional irritant dermatitis. A child who makes himself filthy at play will need a bath, but the general advice is regular washing but bathing only 2–3 times a week for the dry-skinned eczema child; a child with eczema may enjoy his bath however, so that the number of baths a week will vary from individual to individual. Skin cleansing by short contact with soap may benefit eczema[5], perhaps by removing bacteria and other debris and allowing topical applications to be more effective: However, soap substitutes should be equally beneficial and less liable to irritate eczematous skin. Contact, as in kissing or bathing, with sufferers from herpes simplex with active cold sores, must be avoided because the individual with eczema may acquire widespread simplex *(eczema herpeticum)* and can become very ill; eczema herpeticum (Figure 3.11) is usually a manifestation of primary herpes infection.

Topical applications include preparations containing tar such as zinc and coal tar paste applied directly to the skin and then covered with cotton bandages or elasticated tubular stockinette. Prescribable occlusive impregnated bandages such as zinc paste and coal tar bandage covered with cotton bandages may be used over the limbs, and parents can be instructed in their application.

Topical hydrocortisone alone or in combination with tar, an antiseptic, or an antibiotic is of benefit and I find a combination of tar and hydrocortisone the most effective. Hydrocortisone is very useful to combat itching, and an antiseptic or antibiotic in combination with it will help to counteract secondary infection. Mupirocin is a valuable topical antibiotic for infected eczema and can be used alone in the short-term when infection has flared the eczema or at the same time as a topical steroid; unfortunately, mupirocin-resistant strains of *Staphylococcus aureus* are appearing[6]. If a topical steroid is used, it should be preferably hydrocortisone ointment or hydrocortisone cream, but in any case as weak a preparation as will control the itching and eruption adequately. Other mildly potent topical steroids are fluocinolone acetonide (0.0025%) and alclometasone dipropionate.

Moderately potent steroids and drug combinations containing steroids are useful for more severe eczema and they include clobetasone butyrate and a combination of clobetasone butyrate, nystatin, and oxytetracycline. Urea promotes hydration of the skin and is useful alone as a 10% cream or combined with hydrocortisone. Most of the children referred to my clinics do not require the potent or very potent topical steroid preparations that they have often already received, and their eczema can be reasonably controlled with the weaker preparations. Potent steroids, e.g. betamethasone valerate, are sometimes necessary, of course, but should be reserved for use sparingly, infrequently, and in the short-term only, over more severely affected areas, because of their well-known topical and even systemic side effects. Occasionally, systemic corticosteroids or adrenocorticotrophic hormone (ACTH) may be required in acute severe uncontrolled atopic dermatitis: short-term treatment should be the aim.

Antihistamines in a dose sufficient to allay itching are useful by day and at night, and short-term dosage may be of adult proportions if itching is severe. It is important to remember that the affected individual often scratches during sleep. In atopic eczema itching is the main problem and it is the itch that requires treatment. Trimeprazine or hydroxyzine hydrochloride are particularly useful. One problem I have found with promethazine hydrochloride is that it may produce unwanted euphoria in the young child. Other sedative antihistamines I find helpful are chlorpheniramine maleate, brompheniramine maleate, and clemastine fumarate. The newer non-sedative antihistamines, terfenadine and astemizole are not of help in atopic eczema.

Systemic antibiotic treatment should be prescribed for severe secondary bacterial infection of the skin, and clearing of such infection may sometimes improve the eczema where infection has been the cause of an exacerbation. Oral evening primrose oil, providing γ-linolenic acid, may improve atopic eczema.

Wearing cotton gloves or mittens to prevent scratching and secondary infection is important and also allows healing of affected hands treated with ointment. Keeping fingernails clean and short is also essential. Sunlight and ultraviolet light are generally beneficial, although the condition of a few children undoubtedly worsens with such exposure. Severe intractable eczema is an indication to admit to hospital for a period of treatment, both for the patient's sake and to relieve the strain on long-suffering parents. The move from home itself is often beneficial to the patient, but I believe that, in general, the child should have a short-term stay of 1–3 weeks, aiming both to clear the eczema and also to indicate to parents how to control it similarly at home. Hospital stay also allows an assessment of both affected individual and parents, and this can be very useful in future management.

Diet, allergy, and atopic eczema

Environmental influences on eczema include diet, inhalants, infections, climate, weather, and personal relationships at home and outside. Food intolerance, whether allergic or otherwise, is occasionally of some importance in children. Inhalants, such as house dust, seem to be of greater importance in the older individual.

Repeated ingestion of a dietary allergen may result in the development of allergy and the occurrence of a diffuse erythematous rash[7], vomiting, urticaria, or even anaphylaxis. Urticaria is not atopic eczema, and any atopic eczema already present may not necessarily worsen with exposure to the allergen than produces urticaria. The widespread itching that accompanies urticaria however, will possibly tend to make existing eczema more itchy and thus more prone to scratching, and may tend to localize atopic eczema occurring later to the most irritant areas[8].

It has been suggested that after a time or with repeated exposure an allergen initially producing an erythema or urticaria in the atopic patient ceases to cause urticaria but sets off itching and scratching manifesting as eczema[9]. In practice, however, it is unusual to find atopic eczema starting other than *per se*, and this perhaps offers some evidence in favour of immediate hypersensitivity to dietary allergens playing no great part in the pathogenesis of atopic eczema. Atopic eczema can, of course, worsen with an allergen that does not produce urticaria.

In a review of many studies evidence favoured the hypothesis that giving infants cow's milk or solids increases the risk of allergic disease[10]. In a large study reported over 50 years ago the incidence of infantile eczema was lowest in breast-fed infants[11]. Exclusive breast feeding is to be encouraged particularly in the first three months of life, as it may delay the onset of atopic eczema in some predisposed children. However, atopic eczema is not uncommon even while the child is still being wholly breast fed and a recent paper from Helsinki[12], indicated that prolonged breast feeding did not prevent atopy; some such babies developing eczema may be sensitized by foods eaten by their mothers[13] and maternal dietary exclusion particularly of eggs and cow's milk seems to benefit some breast-fed babies with eczema[14]. Nutritionally complete soya protein-containing cow's milk substitutes, prescribable as borderline substances, may benefit some children with atopic eczema if there is good evidence of milk-protein allergy, and the history from the mother, including any mention of gastrointestinal symptoms, is important. It should not be forgotten that allergy to soya can also develop, and a recent infant study found soya feeds to be associated with eczema as often as cow's milk-based feeds[15]. Occasionally, boiled or long-life milk can be tolerated while raw milk cannot, perhaps because denatured proteins are not so allergenic as natural ones. Food intolerance proved in infancy may resolve in many cases with age.

The substitution of goat's milk for cow's milk is unlikely to be beneficial and is not recommended for infants. It has certain dangers such as a high solute load, and deficiency of folic acid and probably vitamins B_{12}, C and D. Furthermore, untreated goat's milk should not be fed to young babies because of the risk of bacterial infection, which in practice is usually introduced by those handling the milk.

An elimination diet is followed for a period of four to six weeks, and, for example, all cow's milk, eggs, beef, fish and chicken are excluded, and then each of these items is reintroduced separately into the diet. Such a diet should be carefully supervised by a dietetic department in conjunction with a dermatologist or paediatrician. Even so, compliance is a real problem in children when they go to birthday parties and so on. Other elimination diets may exclude only milk and eggs or wheat or fruits, or benzoate preservatives and colouring agents such as tartrazine. There is obvious wisdom in withdrawing suspect harmful foods, but reintroduction should be carried out in hospital, if possible, because of the danger of anaphylaxis[16]. Oral sodium cromoglycate may also have a place when food allergy is suspected.

If house-dust mites are considered a factor in worsening of atopic eczema then spraying of bedding with natamycin may be indicated. This spray reduces the *Aspergillus* population (an important food source for the house-dust mite); extra thorough vacuuming in all living rooms can be just as effective, and an inexpensive air purifier may also help. It is also worth noting that furry toys accumulate dust.

It must always be remembered that atopic eczema is subject to spontaneous exacerbations and remissions and claims for any particular treatment must always be assessed with this in mind.

Further points

The medical social worker can have an important role to play in the management of atopic eczema, particularly in assessing the family background[17]. An unhappy child often shows unhappy skin (dry, rubbed, excoriated), or he may wheeze. Overcrowded home or school conditions may lead to worsening of eczema and indicate a need for rehousing or a change of school. Atopic eczema is not a contraindication either for diphtheria, tetanus and pertussis inoculation or for oral polio vaccine.

Those with active eczema should avoid occupations such as engineering (which involves contact with irritant chemicals such as oils and degreasing agents), hairdressing, and similar occupations. Atopic eczema tends to improve with age, a point one always emphasizes to parents, but it is impossible to prophesy the prognosis in a particular child: 50% of children are clear by the age of 6 years, and 90% are clear by the age of 15 years. In some, however, eczema will reappear later on, and this emphasizes the importance of long-term follow up when one talks of prognosis in atopic eczema[18, 19].

As a group, children with eczema tend to be bright and intelligent. Many healthy atopics in families of average height are of short stature for their chronological age, but they usually shoot up around puberty and beyond. Parents should be instructed to allow an affected child to lead a normal life and not allow him to rule the roost to the detriment of siblings or to direct their lives. For instance, children with eczema should neither be permitted to share the nuptial bed nor be bribed to stop scratching; a parent must not yield to the child who threatens to scratch if he is not given what he wants. I emphasize that firmness with love is an important rule in the correct management of the young atopic.

Atopic eczema is a common problem and its treatment requires the patience and cooperation of family, patient, family practitioner, and with more severely affected children, the dermatologist and social worker.

JUVENILE PLANTAR DERMATOSIS

This is a frictional dermatitis (Figure 3.14) seen frequently in the 0–17 years' group in which itching and burning occur over the plantar aspect of the big toes and then spread to the other toes and the whole forefoot. The heel may be affected but to a lesser degree. The affected forefoot becomes red, glazed, dry, cracked, sore and painful and there is often peeling and bleeding. The child may have difficulty in walking. Toe spaces are notably unaffected. The condition may persist for a number of years. The disorder was first observed in the 1960s and there is little doubt that synthetic footwear with little or absent permeability and poor moisture absorption is an important factor in the aetiology. I and others[20] believe atopics to be prone to this condition, but it is also common in non-atopics. Cotton socks, leather shoes, urea-containing creams and yellow soft paraffin have a place in management.

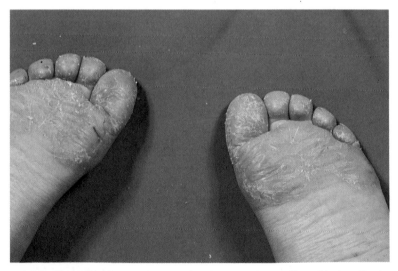

Figure 3.14 **Juvenile plantar dermatosis.** Note the dry peeling skin localized to the forefoot in this atopic boy of 7 years.

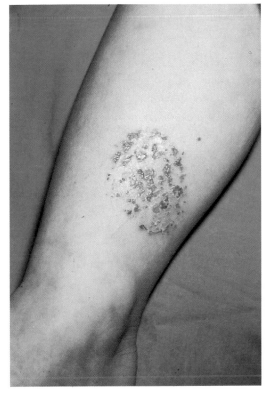

Figure 3.15 **Nummular eczema.** Impetiginized lesion over leg.

NUMMULAR ECZEMA

This condition (Figure 3.15) in children is often a manifestation of atopy. Coin-shaped lesions which tend to be symmetrical are seen primarily over the limbs. Secondary bacterial infection of lesions is common. Nummular eczema has a tendency to be recurrent and chronic.

LICHEN STRIATUS

This is an uncommon asymptomatic self-limiting, usually unilateral dermatitis of unknown origin, seen in children and young adults (Figures 3.16 and 3.17). Lichenoid papules appear, usually over a limb and extend in a linear manner over a period of days or weeks. There may be slight scaling associated. Differential diagnosis includes an epidermal naevus, psoriasis, and linear lichen planus.

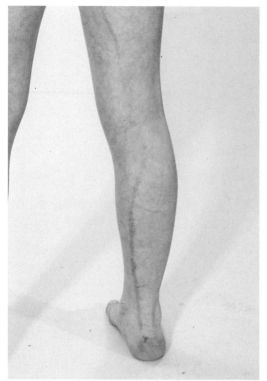

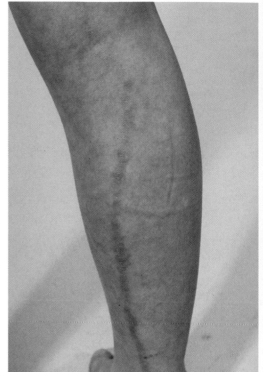

Figure 3.16 **Lichen striatus** over a lower limb in a 7-year-old girl.

Figure 3.17 **Lichen striatus.** Close-up of leg lesion.

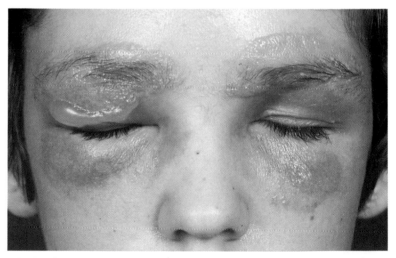

Figure 3.18 **Contact dermatitis** in a boy of 13 years. He had applied various antiseptics around the eyes and then erythema and blistering followed. Allergic contact dermatitis was considered likely but no cause was found.

CONTACT DERMATITIS

Irritant dermatitis

This indicates a non-allergic reaction of the skin. The child with atopic dermatitis is prone to such contact dermatitis. Napkin dermatitis is mentioned in Chapter 5.

Allergic dermatitis

This is a manifestation of delayed hypersensitivity to a contact allergen and the eruption always occurs initially at the site of skin contact with the allergen (Figure 3.18). If contact dermatitis is suspected by the distribution and appearance of skin lesions, patch testing should always be performed. However, in my experience allergic dermatitis is uncommon under the age of 12 years.

Photosensitive dermatitis

In this condition (Figure 3.19) some substances are transformed into primary irritants or sensitizers after light exposure and a dermatitis can result; such reactions may be phototoxic (e.g. tars and certain plants) or photoallergic (e.g. perfumes).

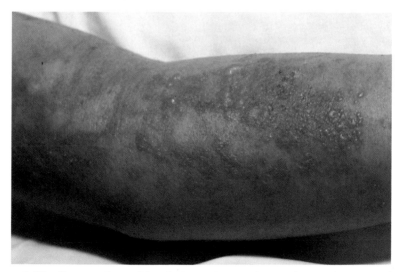

Figure 3.19 **Contact dermatitis of arm—phototoxic reaction.** An acute vesicular dermatitis occurred in this girl of 8 years following sun exposure after removal of a tar-impregnated cotton bandage (applied because of atopic dermatitis).

REFERENCES

1. Merrett, J., Barnetson, R. St. C., Burr, M. L. and Merrett, T. G. (1984). Total and specific IgG4 antibody levels in atopic eczema. *Clin. Exp. Immunol.* **56**, 645–52
2. Colver, G. B., Mortimer, P. S., Millard, P. R., Dawber, R. P. R. and Ryan, T. J. (1987). The 'dirty neck'—a reticulate pigmentation in atopics. *Clin. Exp. Dermatol.*, **12**, 1–4
3. Finn, R., Harvey, M. M., Johnson, P. M., Verbov, J. L. and Barnes, R. M. R. (1985). Serum IgG antibodies to gliadin and other dietary antigens in adults with atopic eczema. *Clin. Exp. Dermatol.*, **10**, 222–8
4. Lessof, M. H. (1983). Food intolerance and allergy—a review. *Q. J. Med.*, **206**, 111–19
5. Uehara, M and Tekada, K. (1985). Use of soap in the management of atopic dermatitis. *Clin. Exp. Dermatol.*, **10**, 419–25
6. Rahman, M., Noble, W. C. and Cookson, B. (1987). Mupirocin-resistant *Staphylococcus aureus. Lancet,* **2**, 387. Also Baird, D. and Coia, J. (1987). Mupirocin-resistant *Staphylococcus aureus. Lancet,* **2**, 387–8
7. Sampson, H. A. and Jolie, P. L. (1984). Increased plasma histamine concentrations after food challenges in children with atopic dermatitis. *N. Engl. J. Med.*, **311**, 372–6
8. Verbov, J. (1985). Elimination diets in eczema. *Arch. Dis. Child.*, **60**, 183–4
9. Sampson, H. A. (1988). Role of immediate food hypersensitivity in the pathogenesis of atopic dermatitis. *J. Allergy Clin. Immunol.*, **71**, 473–80
10. Burr, M. L. (1983). Does infant feeding affect the risk of allergy? *Arch. Dis. Child.*, **58**, 561–5
11. Grulee, C. G. and Sanford, H. N. (1936). The influence of breast and artificial feeding on infantile eczema. *J. Pediatr.*, **89**, 223–5
12. Savilahti, E., Tainio, V-M., Salmenpera, L., Siimes, M. A. and Perheentupa, J. (1987). Prolonged exclusive breast feeding and heredity as determinants in infantile atopy. *Arch. Dis. Child.*, **62**, 269–73
13. Cant, A., Marsden, R. A. and Kilshaw, P. J. (1985). Egg and cows' milk hypersensitivity in exclusively breast fed infants with eczema and detection of egg protein in breast milk. *Br. Med. J.*, **291**, 932–5
14. Cant, A. J., Bailes, J. A., Marsden, R. A. and Hewitt, D. (1986). Effect of maternal dietary exclusion on breast-fed infants with eczema: two controlled studies. *Br. Med. J.*, **293**, 231–3
15. Moore, W. J., Midwinter, R. E., Morris, A. F., Colley, J. R. J. and Soothill, J. F. (1985). Infant feeding and subsequent risk of atopic eczema. *Arch. Dis. Child.*, **60**, 722–6
16. David, T. J. (1984). Anaphylactic shock during elimination diets for severe atopic eczema. *Arch. Dis. Child.*, **59**, 983–6
17. McSkimming, J., Gleeson, L. and Sinclair, M. (1984). A pilot study of a support group for parents of children with eczema. *Aust. J. Dermatol.*, **25**, 8–11
18. Vickers, C. F. H. (1980). The natural history of atopic eczema. *Acta Dermatol. Venereol. (Stockh.),* suppl. **92**, 113–15
19. Rystedt, I. (1985). Prognostic factors in atopic dermatitis. *Acta Dermatol. Venereol. (Stockh.),* **65**, 206–13
20. Jones, S. K., English, J. S. C., Forsyth, A. and MacKie, R. M. (1987). Juvenile plantar dermatosis—an 8-year follow-up of 102 patients. *Clin. Exp. Dermatol.*, **12**, 5–7

4

Infections and Infestations

CONTENTS

Flea bites
Papular urticaria
Creeping eruption (cutaneous larva migrans)
Cutaneous leishmaniasis (oriental sore)

BACTERIAL INFECTIONS

Impetigo

Impetigo (Figures 4.1 and 4.2) occurs mainly in children and its occurrence in the newborn as bullous impetigo has been mentioned (Chapter 2). It is usually due to *Staphylococcus aureus* but may be complicated by *Streptococcus*. It is often associated with poor hygienic conditions and rapidly spreads among members of the household. Flaccid blisters appear, few or many, most commonly

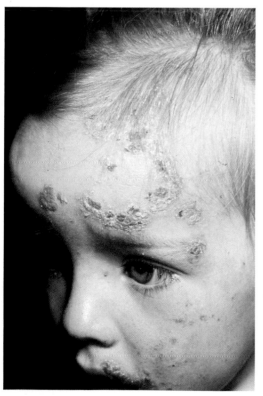

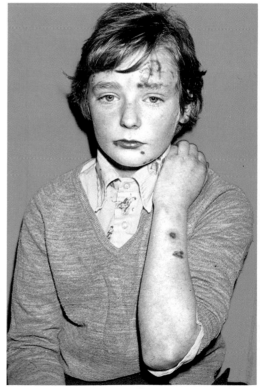

Figure 4.1 **Impetigo.** Crusted lesions are visible in this boy of 2 years.

Figure 4.2 **Impetigo.** Facial and forearm lesions.

over the face, and these quickly dry and crust. Lesions may also be ringed with a crusted edge. In treatment, removal of crusts is important because bacteria are present in the lesions and infected crusts encourage spread of impetigo. After removal of crusts, application of antiseptic or antibiotic ointment such as fusidic acid, aureomycin, or mupirocin, is indicated. If impetigo is widespread or haemolytic streptococci are present, a full course of an oral antibiotic is indicated and this may help to prevent the occasional complication of acute glomerulonephritis following streptococcal impetigo. More common than impetigo itself is impetiginization of other conditions such as eczema, scabies, head-lice infestation, papular urticaria, herpes simplex and herpes zoster, often encouraged by inappropriate use of topical corticosteroids.

Ecthyma

This is of similar causation to impetigo. Lesions are often multiple and occur particularly over lower limbs. They have adherent crusts with underlying ulceration. Affected children are often debilitated or malnourished.

Staphylococcal scalded skin syndrome

This is seen (Figures 4.3 and 4.4) usually in the under-five age group has already been mentioned in Chapter 2. It may be preceded by a purulent conjunctivitis, otitis media, or an upper respiratory infection. Staphylococci can be isolated from such foci and there may be a history of typical impetigo in a sibling. There may be widespread skin involvement but mucosae are unaffected. Pustules are rare in this condition except in the napkin and periumbilical areas of neonates. Recovery without scarring is usually within 5–7 days with or without antibiotics, but I feel it is safer to treat all cases with penicillinase-resistant penicillin or fusidic acid.

Cellulitis

Erysipelas is an acute cellulitis due to Group A haemolytic streptococci entering through a break in the skin usually near the eye, ear, nostril or mouth. Low-grade facial cellulitis is much more common and may be recurrent. Sites of entry are as for erysipelas. When attacks of cellulitis are recurrent there is often an underlying defect of lymph drainage in the affected areas and such patients may show

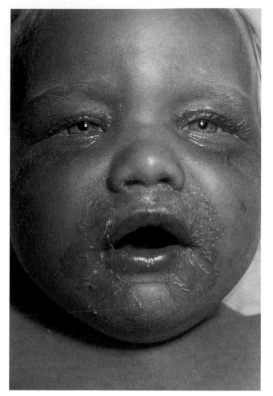

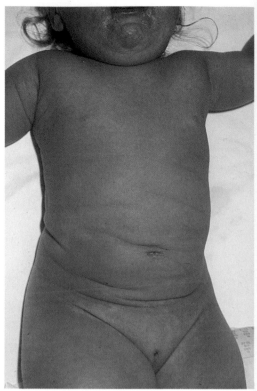

Figure 4.3 **Staphylococcal scalded skin syndrome.** This 1-year-old child showed a generalized erythema. This close-up shows eyelid and perioral involvement.

Figure 4.4 **Staphylococcal scalded skin syndrome.** Same child as in Figure 4.3 showing her widespread erythema.

persistent residual lymphoedema associated with tissue fibrosis after recurrent attacks. Although usually due to haemolytic streptococcal infection, cellulitis can be caused by other organisms such as *Staphylococcus aureus, Streptococcus pneumoniae* and *Haemophilus influenzae.*

Meninogococcaemia

This is seen particularly in pre-school children and may present with purpuric lesions which are most common over trunk and lower limbs (Figures 4.5 and 4.6). In severe infections, large ecchymotic areas with sharply-defined borders may be seen; lesions result from both intravascular coagulation and bacterial damage to blood vessels.

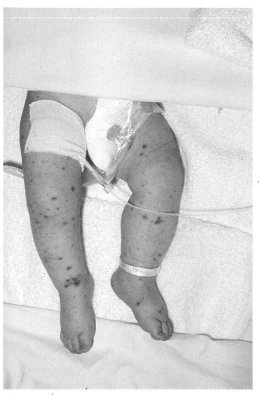

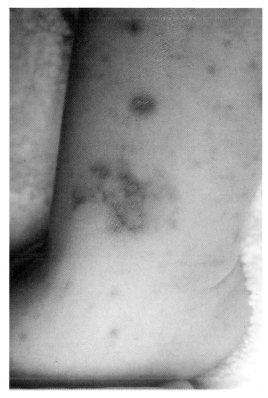

Figure 4.5 **Meningococcaemia.** A 7-month-old baby with purpura over the legs.

Figure 4.6 **Meningococcaemia.** Close-up showing purpura and necrotic lesions.

VIRAL INFECTIONS

Warts

Warts (Figure 4.7) are caused by a DNA-containing papillomavirus with over forty types identified and these infect and replicate in skin and mucosa. Warts, of course, are very common, particularly in children and young adults, with fingers and soles being the usual sites, although knees and face are also common sites. In children, virtually all warts disappear spontaneously within three years and many disappear within months rather than years. Warts are uncommon under the age of 3 years. Patients receiving corticosteroid or cytotoxic therapy and those with atopic dermatitis are more susceptible to the wart virus. Warts are not usually painful but if they are it usually indicates that secondary infection is present, or in the case of plantar warts

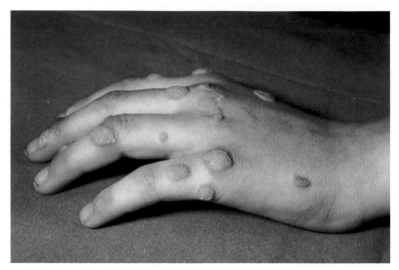

Figure 4.7 **Warts.** Typical florid finger warts.

(verrucae), it is the overlying callosity that is painful on pressure over the affected area. Reassurance is the best treatment for warts but treatment includes use of liquid nitrogen cryotherapy or nightly application of salicylic acid (12%) in collodion (to 100%) for finger warts, and peeling applications containing salicylic acid such as salicylic acid (16.7%), lactic acid (16.7%) in collodion (to 100%) to plantar warts. Plantar warts are no reason for denying swimming and affected children should be free to enter a pool with their warts covered by a waterproof plaster, or wearing lightweight shoe socks of which there are many types. A 5–15% podophyllin in tinct. benzoin co. can be applied to perianal or vulval warts but the area of application should be washed 4–6 hours later. Management of warts has been discussed in a recent symposium[1].

Molluscum contagiosum

This is due to a pox virus and the infection is common in infants and children (Figures 4.8 and 4.9). Lesions may be single but are usually multiple and appear as discrete pearly papules often with central umbilication; occasionally giant, usually solitary lesions occur. Multiple lesions are common in children with atopic dermatitis and are encouraged by the use of topical steroids. It is interesting that some children, whether atopic or not, show eczema in an area of mollusca. The ano-genital region, trunk and face are common sites but they can

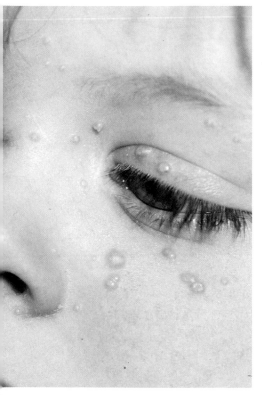

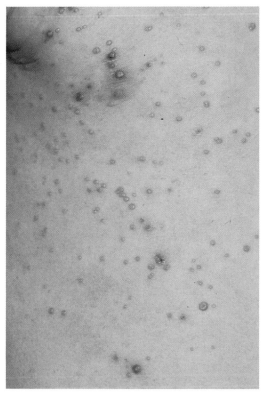

Figure 4.8 **Molluscum contagiosum.** Some of the pearly lesions show umbilication.

Figure 4.9 **Molluscum contagiosum.** Widespread in an atopic dermatitis sufferer. Note the Köbner phenomenon in one area (see psoriasis in Chapter 5).

appear anywhere. Parents should be reassured that the lesions are benign and will disappear spontaneously within a year without therapy. Resolution of lesions is sometimes hastened by secondary bacterial infection, but such lesions are more likely to leave residual superficial scarring.

Herpes simplex

The primary infection with herpes simplex (Figures 4.10 and 4.11) usually presents as herpetic stomatitis between the ages of 1–4 years. It presents as fever with mouth ulceration often with a few vesicles over the lips, or as a sore throat. The condition usually resolves spontaneously over a period of a week or so, but symptomatic treatment may be necessary in more severe cases. Although genital infections are

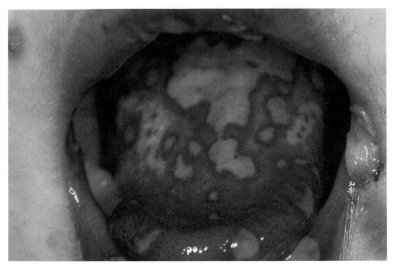

Figure 4.10 **Herpes simplex.** Severe erosive stomatitis in a 5-year-old. This is primary infection.

usually caused by Type II virus, female infants are occasionally seen with herpes vulvo-vaginitis, due to Type I virus, transmitted by touch, either from their own herpes stomatitis or from another's cold sores.

Secondary herpes infection (Figures 4.12 and 4.13) is commonly recurrent and presents in older children as grouped vesicles on a red background, usually over the face. Vesicles burst, dry, and crust

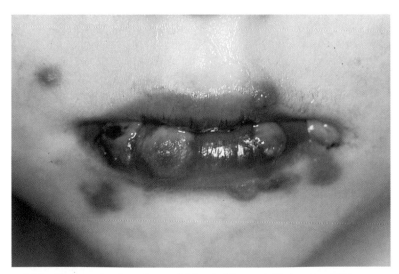

Figure 4.11 **Herpes simplex.** Same child as in Figure 4.10 showing blisters over lips.

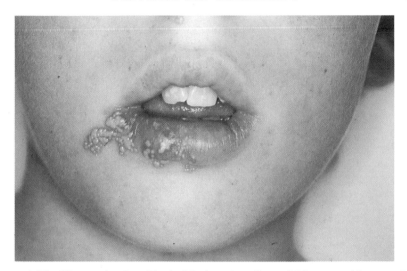

Figure 4.12 **Herpes simplex.** Typical lesions in a boy of 10 years with secondary simplex infection. The lesions appeared during the course of meningococcal meningitis.

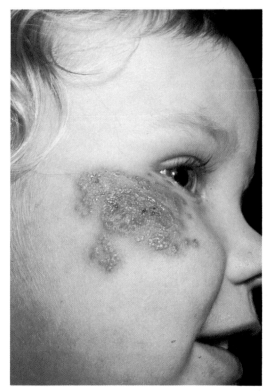

Figure 4.13 **Herpes simplex.** Secondary (recurrent) simplex in a boy of 3½ years; he is young to have secondary simplex.

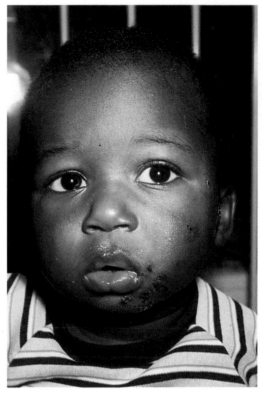

Figure 4.14 **Herpes zoster.** Here affecting left trigeminal nerve, showing involvement of left side of chin, cheek, scalp and anterior to pinna in a Nigerian infant of 1 year. His mother had varicella when 8 months pregnant with him, and he would have first been exposed to the varicella-zoster virus at that time.

within about ten days. Known precipitating factors are exposure to sun, cold, menstruation and fever. Topical acyclovir cream is useful in treatment.

Herpes zoster

This acute infection (Figure 4.14) is caused by the varicella virus and an attack is due to reactivation of this virus in the individual. The eruption of groups of vesicles on an erythematous background is unilateral over one or more dermatomes. Vesicles may erupt for a few weeks and secondary infection of lesions is common. Symptoms are usually mild in prepubertal children but a severe attack merits systemic acyclovir; use of the topical application to intact vesicles is routine.

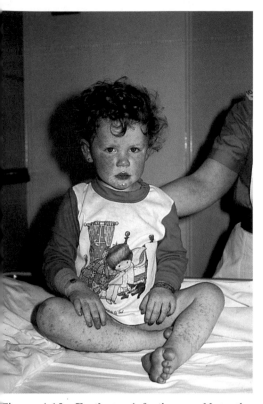 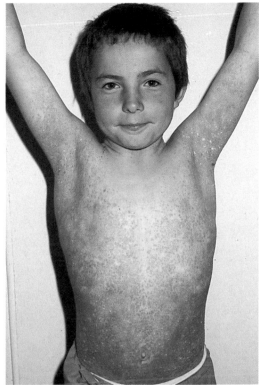

Figure 4.15 **Erythema infectiosum.** Note the slapped-cheek appearance and the early maculo-papular rash over the limbs.

Figure 4.16 **Erythema infectiosum.** Maculo-papular erythematous trunk lesions in a 9-year-old boy. His two brothers also had the infection.

Erythema infectiosum (fifth disease)

This is due to human parvovirus B-19 and small outbreaks of the condition are not uncommon, particularly in the spring (Figures 4.15–4.17). The incubation period is 7–10 days. Rose-red papules on the cheeks become confluent, giving a slapped-cheek appearance. During the next few days, erythematous maculo-papules appear over the limbs and trunk, often developing into a lace-like (reticular) pattern. The latter eruption usually fades within 10 days but may reappear. In most children, systemic symptoms are usually minimal. Arthritis is sometimes a complication but more particularly in adults.

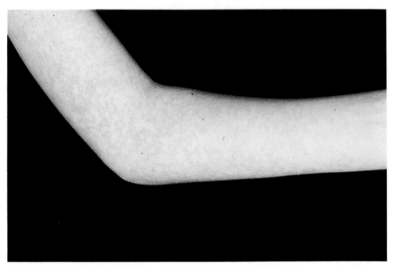

Figure 4.17 **Erythema infectiosum.** An 8-year-old boy. Note the net-like erythema. His twin brother was also affected. Both had minimal symptoms starting with red cheeks two weeks previously.

Hand, foot and mouth disease

This affects children particularly (Figure 4.18), and has usually been associated with a Coxsackie virus and less commonly Enterovirus 71. The disease is commonly mild, lasting about seven days and with an incubation period of 5–7 days. It presents with a painful stomatitis

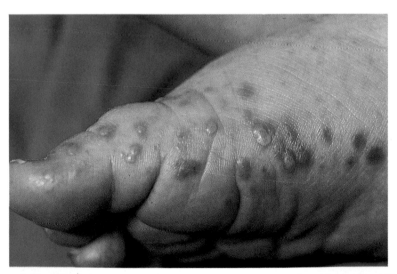

Figure 4.18 **Hand, foot and mouth disease.** Blisters over foot in a 14-month-old boy.

with superficial small flaccid blisters visible over the buccal mucosa. Similar vesicles, which may vary in size, occur over hands and feet and a maculo-papular rash may appear over the buttocks. If in close contact whole families are often affected.

Gianotti-Crosti syndrome (papular acrodermatitis of childhood)

This self-limiting dermatosis (Figure 4.19) is characterized by the sudden onset of coppery-red non-pruritic lichenoid papules over face, buttocks and extremities, but sparing the trunk. There may be a purpuric appearance to lesions. Constitutional symptoms are usually

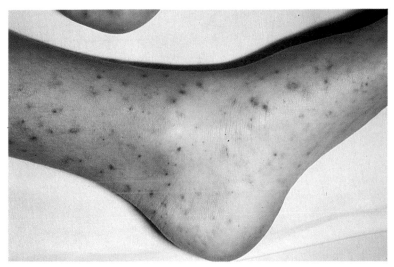

Figure 4.19 **Gianotti-Crosti syndrome.** Red papular lesions over lower leg. Lethargy and anorexia preceded the rash. His liver enzyme levels were elevated early on in the disorder.

mild but there may be anicteric hepatitis, hepatomegaly, and widespread lymphadenopathy. The main age range for incidence of this syndrome is 1–6 years. The disorder is probably viral in origin and hepatitis B antigen has been reported in some cases: Coxsackie, Epstein–Barr, and parainfluenza viruses may produce the same disorder[2].

Human immunodeficiency virus (HIV) infection

Children acquire HIV infection[3] *in utero* or perinatally, or by receiving contaminated blood products. The cutaneous manifestations are primarily fungal, bacterial or viral infections. Persistent oral candidiasis occurs frequently and widespread seborrhoeic dermatitis may be seen. Vasculitis and thrombocytopenic purpura are among other complications.

FUNGAL INFECTIONS

Candidiasis

Oral candidiasis is common in the newborn and can also affect older children. Patches of adherent white material are seen scattered over the mucous membrane. In the newborn the organism is usually derived from the maternal vagina. Perianal candidiasis may follow spread of the organism through the bowel. Napkin area eruptions associated with candidial infection are mentioned in Chapter 5 and chronic paronychia in Chapter 6.

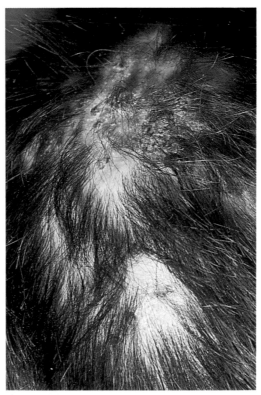

Figure 4.20   **Ringworm.** *Trichophyton violaceum* (an anthropophilic fungus) was cultured from scalp hairs in this 3-year-old Bangladeshi child domiciled in England. Affected areas healed without scarring.

Chronic mucocutaneous candidiasis is a rare condition with many causes; it affects mouth and nails particularly. Candidal granuloma of the scalp indicates hyperkeratotic areas of candidiasis, in children showing a variety of immunological abnormalities.

Ringworm

Ringworm infection (Figures 4.20–4.23) may affect hair, skin and nails and infection is acquired from other humans (i.e. anthropophilic), animals (i.e. zoophilic), or from the soil (i.e. geophilic). Scalp ringworm (tinea capitis) is common but tinea cruris and chronic nail infection (tinea unguium) are uncommon in children. Cattle ringworm (*Trichophyton verrucosum*) can give rise to markedly inflammatory red patches covered with pustules (kerion) but ringworm

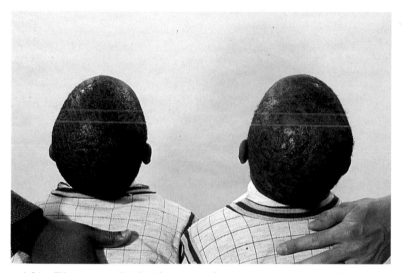

Figure 4.21 **Ringworm.** *Trichophyton soudanense* (an anthropophilic fungus) was cultured from these 6-year-old twin girls. Hair fall appeared in England four months after leaving Nigeria. These girls were kept away from school because of risk of spreading infection to other children; they returned to school after contacts were screened and the twins were non-infective.

infections from cats and dogs (*Microsporum canis*) tend to produce less marked inflammation, although kerion can occur, and are characterized in the scalp by hair loss and broken-off hairs with a varying degree of erythema and scaling. Hairs infected with *Microsporum audouinii* (an anthropophilic fungus) or *M. canis*

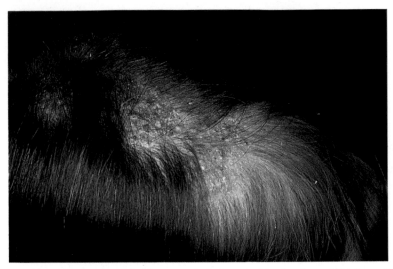

Figure 4.22 **Ringworm.** This illustrates hair loss and kerion in a child from North Wales whose dog also had ringworm (*M. canis*). This child with a zoophilic infection, would not require exclusion from school because infectivity from human to human is only slight.

fluoresce green under a Wood's light and this is a useful mass-screening procedure. The circular lesions of tinea corporis are easily identified by their active raised scaling margins. Tinea pedis is commonly seen, manifested by interdigital scaling or acute blister

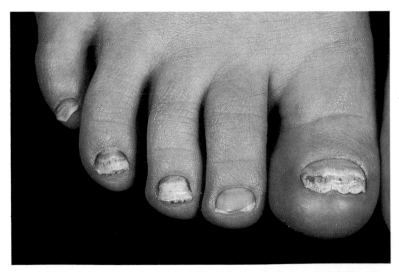

Figure 4.23 **Ringworm.** Thickened discoloured toe nails infected with *T. rubrum* are shown in a boy of 3½ years with abnormal nails present since he was 8 months old. He received treatment with oral griseofulvin and topical imidazoles.

formation. In ringworm infection of nails, the feet of family members should be examined because the source will often be found and adults affected should be treated more vigorously. Big toenails are particularly affected, being thickened, irregular and white or yellowish in colour.

A diagnosis of ringworm can be confirmed by observing fungal filaments in microscopic preparations softened with potassium hydroxide, but culture is required to identify the particular fungus concerned. In treating ringworm, use a topical imidazole preparation alone or sometimes in conjunction with oral griseofulvin; the latter should be taken for 4–6 weeks in skin or hair infection and for 6–18 months for nail ringworm.

Pityriasis versicolor

This is a superficial fungus infection caused by a *Pityrosporum* yeast. It is most common in young adults but does occur in older children. Scaling patches appear particularly over the upper trunk and upper arms. Lesions may be hypopigmented or hyperpigmented. It is often asymptomatic but some patients, particularly those from warmer climes, do itch. Application of selenium sulphide (2.5%) in liquid shampoo form at bedtime, washed off next morning and repeated one week later is usually effective. An imidazole cream applied twice daily for three weeks is an alternative treatment.

PARASITIC INFESTATIONS

Scabies

Human scabies Human scabies (Figures 4.24–4.28) is due to *Sarcoptes scabiei* var. *hominis* and presents after an incubation period of 2–6 weeks following infestation with the mite with burrows over the finger and toe spaces, front of wrists, breasts, axillary folds, buttocks, backs of elbows and penis. In infants, and they may be as young as 5–6 weeks old, the eruption is often even more widespread, sometimes with firm papules or nodules over the trunk, and papules, vesico-papules or pustules over palms and soles; burrows are not always visible. Excoriations, eczematized and impetiginized lesions are frequent and a secondary sensitization eruption of urticarial type may complicate the infestation. Incidentally, in hot humid climates, absence of burrows is a regular finding in scabies[4]. Scabies is

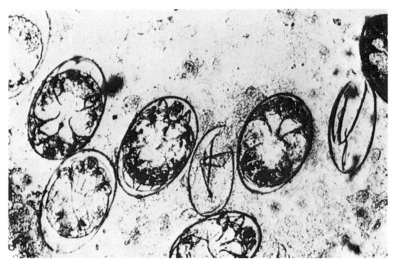

Figure 4.24   **Scabies.** Photograph of scraping of burrow showing numerous larvae and empty egg cases.

common and it is most important that it should be remembered in the differential diagnosis of irritant dermatoses; it is often forgotten. If using lindane lotion or cream as treatment, because of possible CNS toxicity with repeated application, this should be applied once only without a preceding bath, to all areas below the face and left on for

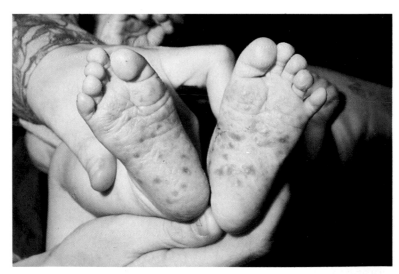

Figure 4.25   **Scabies.** In infants, papules, pustules and vesicles affecting the soles are common.

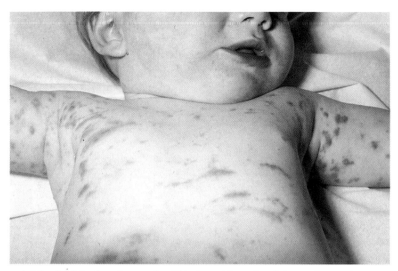

Figure 4.26 **Scabies** in a 9-month-old baby with urticarial reaction and eczematization of some lesions. He had had scabies since the age of 4 months.

8–12 hours. All members of the family in contact, whether symptomatic or not, should be treated. Other treatments include 25% benzyl benzoate emulsion which is applied below the face to all areas and repeated 24 hours later. Benzyl benzoate tends to sting and must not be applied repeatedly because it is liable to produce an irritant

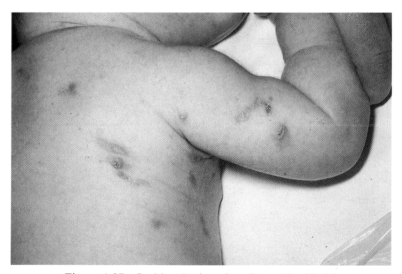

Figure 4.27 **Scabies.** Lesions in a 2-month-old girl.

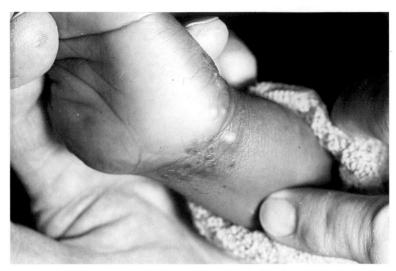

Figure 4.28 **Scabies.** Wrist pustules in a 4-year-old Nigerian child. *Staphylococcus aureus* grew from one of the pustules visible. Scraping was negative for scabies but distribution of eruption and history of other family members with symptoms was important.

dermatitis if so used: It should be applied in one-third strength to infants and one-half strength to children up to the age of 12 years; 0.5% malathion lotion is applied once below the face to all areas and left on for 12 hours; crotamiton lotion or cream is applied twice daily for 5 days; sulphur (6%) in white soft paraffin is applied nightly for three applications. Itching persisting for a few weeks after successful treatment is common and responds to oral antihistamines.

Animal scabies This is due to *Sarcoptes scabiei* var. *canis* and is not uncommon, involving the abdomen, lower chest, thighs and forearms, and there may be facial lesions. It may also be due to *Cheyletiella* species, which are free-living mites in the coats of cats, dogs and rabbits. Pruritus, papules, urticaria or blisters may be seen, particularly prominent at sites of greatest contact with the animal. Lesions usually clear in about three weeks if there is no re-infestation. Treatment of the animal source is indicated.

Lice infestation

This usually presents in children with itching and secondary infection over the nape of the neck. Head lice and nits (egg capsules) will be visible on careful examination. All scalps in the household or classroom should be checked and treated if necessary. Carbaryl shampoo (0.5%) or malathion lotion (0.5%) are recommended preparations, but lindane in a shampoo base still has a place in treatment. Hair cutting is unnecessary. If nits are present on the eyelashes this usually indicates pubic lice infestation acquired from an adult; parents should be discreetly questioned regarding this.

Flea bites

Bites from human, bird, cat, or dog fleas, appear in the young as groups, often linear, of erythematous macular lesions each with a central punctum (Figure 4.29). They are often noticed in the morning on awakening.

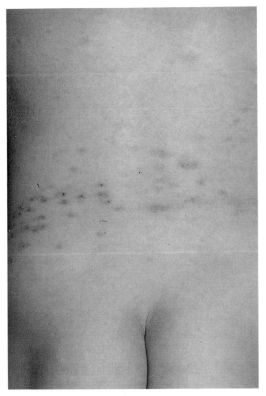

Figure 4.29 **Insect bites.** Flea bites are visible over left hip.

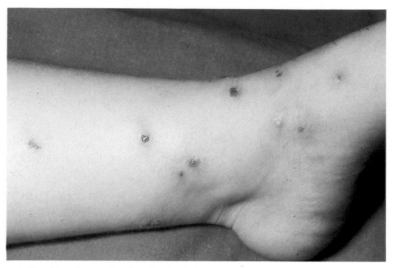

Figure 4.30 **Papular urticaria.** Typical site over leg showing vesicles, some secondarily infected.

Papular urticaria

This is more common than actual insect bites in children. It is rare in the first year of life. It represents a hypersensitivity reaction to a bite from a flea (dog, cat, bird, human), bed bug, mosquito, or dog louse. Irritation, vesicles, papules, and weals appear over buttocks and lower limbs, but distribution may be wider in chronic papular urticaria, and secondary infection of lesions is common (Figure 4.30). Usually only one child in a family shows the urticaria which tends to recur yearly for a few years in the summer. Treatment consists of topical applications such as oily calamine lotion and sometimes oral antihistamines, and pets should be routinely checked for ectoparasites; even the best-kept pets of impeccable pedigree may harbour ectoparasites. Time is well spent explaining the condition to parents.

Creeping eruption (cutaneous larva migrans)

This is a tortuous linear eruption usually caused by larvae of the dog or cat hookworm. Infections are most common in warm, humid and sandy coastal areas of tropical and subtropical regions. The larvae penetrate human skin that has been in contact with contaminated sandy areas and they remain in the skin producing a characteristic serpentine track. Oral mebendazole is used as therapy.

Cutaneous leishmaniasis (oriental sore)

This is an infective granuloma of skin and subcutaneous tissues. The infestation is common among inhabitants of the Mediterranean, Middle East, India and South America and those who travel to these places. The flagellated protozoon parasite (*Leishmania tropica*) is present in juice aspirated from the spreading edge of a sore. The infection is caused by sandflies (*Phlebotomus papatasii*). The incubation period following the bite varies from weeks to many months. An enlarging irritant nodule appears which forms a sore and scab: ulceration may occur in weeks or months. Lesions may be single or multiple. Common sites are the face, legs and arms. Without treatment, healing with a prominent scar usually takes place within a year. Treatment includes removal of crusts and use of antimonials.

REFERENCES

1. Douglass, M. C., Koblenzer, P. J., Moroz, B., Heskel, N. S., Goldberg, G. N., Hurwitz, S., Caputo, R. V. and Boxall, L. (1987). Management of warts in children. *Pediatr. Dermatol.,* **4**, 36–54
2. Spear, K. L. and Winkelmann, R. K. (1984). Gianotti–Crosti syndrome. A review of ten cases not associated with hepatitis B. *Arch. Dermatol.,* **120**, 891–6
3. Prose, N. S., Mendez, H., Menikoff, H. and Miller, H. J. (1987). Pediatric human immunodeficiency virus infection and its cutaneous manifestations. *Pediatr. Dermatol.,* **4**, 67–74
4. Taplin, D., Rivera, A., Graham Walker, J., Roth, W. I., Reno, D. and Meinking, T. (1983). A comparative trial of three treatment schedules for the eradication of scabies. *J. Am. Acad. Dermatol.,* **9**, 550–4

5

Napkin area eruptions and erythemato-squamous disorders

CONTENTS

NAPKIN AREA ERUPTIONS

Napkin (irritant) dermatitis

This is an irritant frictional contact dermatitis and the most common eruption in the napkin area (Figures 5.1–5.3). At least initially, the eruption is most prominent at sites of napkin contact and thus erythema and more severe inflammation will characteristically affect convexities. It usually appears after the first month of life probably

71

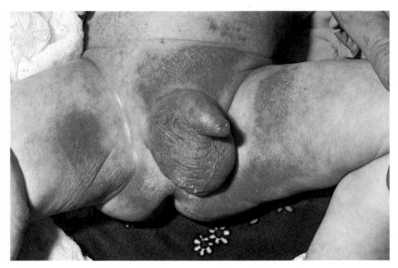

Figure 5.1 **Napkin dermatitis.** W-shaped dermatitis sparing the groins.

because repeated skin insult is required before an eruption becomes obvious. It may occur alone or with other napkin area eruptions. Contact with napkin material soaked in urine irritates the skin of susceptible infants and urea-splitting organisms in faeces or infected urine increases the alkalinity and the likelihood of a dermatitis: Thus, diarrhoea, or soiled napkins left on for prolonged periods encourage

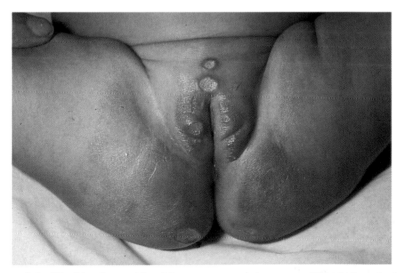

Figure 5.2 **Napkin dermatitis.** More severe erosive type. This infant had an ammoniacal dermatitis.

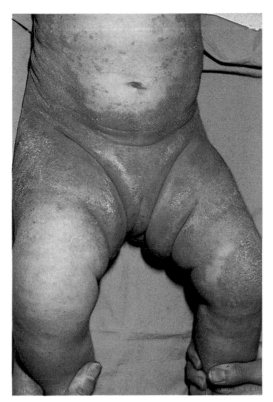

Figure 5.3 **Napkin dermatitis.** Spreading scald appearance over napkin area. *Staphylococcus aureus* complicated the eruption.

the appearance of dermatitis. Regular nappy changing ensures that both urine and faeces spread by the mobile infant do not remain *in situ* for long periods. The modern, more absorbent disposable nappies reducing time of urine contact with the skin are a useful advance. The term *ammoniacal dermatitis* should be correctly applied only to some eroded forms. Treatment of irritant dermatitis is best by exposure if practical. However plastic pants should be avoided and if towelling nappies are normally worn under plastic pants, the wearing of two or three such nappies or a suitable disposable nappy at night will allow plastic pants to be dispensed with. Use of simple emollient or mildly-potent steroid applications is also indicated.

Infantile gluteal granuloma

This is the term describing large erythematous nodules appearing on a background of napkin dermatitis (Figure 5.4). Sometimes their

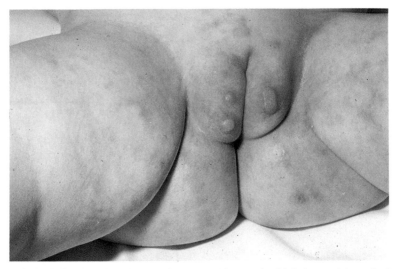

Figure 5.4 **Infantile gluteal granuloma.** A 10-month-old infant with typical soft nodules involving the vulva. The napkin dermatitis is resolving.

appearance may be related to overuse of topical steroids. They resolve spontaneously, but often months after the original napkin dermatitis has resolved.

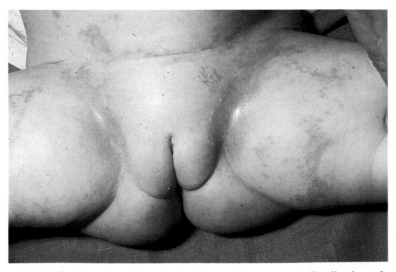

Figure 5.5 **Infantile seborrhoeic dermatitis.** Mild but typical distribution of eruption which began at the age of 2 weeks.

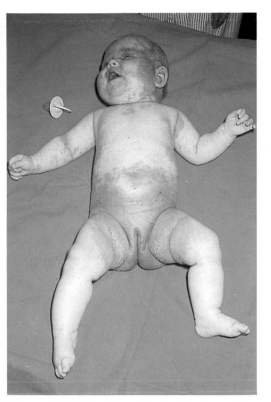 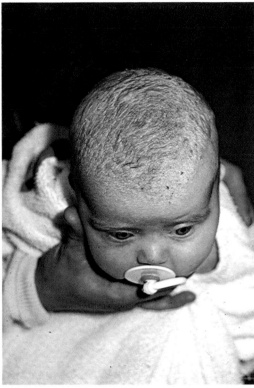

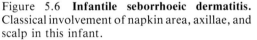

Figure 5.6 **Infantile seborrhoeic dermatitis.** Classical involvement of napkin area, axillae, and scalp in this infant.

Figure 5.7 **Infantile seborrhoeic dermatitis** showing scalp involvement.

Infantile seborrhoeic dermatitis

This condition (Figures 5.5–5.7) is non-irritant and typically occurs within the first three or four months of life and often in the first few weeks, clearing within weeks of onset. The napkin area and particularly the groins, or the scalp, are the common sites of onset but axillae, neck, and post-auricular regions are also usually affected. Erythema, maceration, and scaling involve the skin folds and the adjacent area, but frequently erythema and discrete lesions with greasy-looking scales become more widespread over the trunk and face. Although yellowish greasy scaling of the scalp (cradle cap) may be the only manifestation in some infants, very occasionally infantile seborrhoeic dermatitis can become a generalized erythroderma requiring in-patient management. Local candidal and bacterial infections often complicate infantile seborrhoeic dermatitis and oral candidiasis may also be present. Plastic pants worn over napkins increase the likelihood of secondary infection. Application of topical preparations containing a combination of hydrocortisone and nystatin or an imidazole are useful for napkin involvement. Scalp and forehead can be treated with a cream containing sulphur (2%), salicylic acid (2%) in aqueous cream (to 100%).

Relevant to the cause of seborrhoeic dermatitis may be the fact that under the influence of maternal androgen, there is sebaceous gland activity in the first few months of life. There may be an increased incidence of atopic manifestations appearing later in these children[1], but I consider seborrhoeic dermatitis itself to be a 'sheep in sheep's clothing' and not a manifestation of atopy.

Infantile seborrhoeic dermatitis remains a self-limiting disorder of obscure aetiology and it is likely that *Candida* is merely a secondary invader rather than playing an aetiological role[2]. The relationship, if any, between this condition and seborrhoeic dermatitis in adolescents or adults is unclear.

Napkin psoriasis

Sometimes a napkin area eruption may be psoriasiform with a well-defined edge and with secondary spread over the trunk (Figure 5.8). This is a form of infantile seborrhoeic dermatitis and some have suggested that such children are more likely to develop psoriasis at a later date.

Candidiasis

This presents as a moist erythematous eruption often with satellite pustules, predominantly over buttocks and perianal region (Figure 5.9). Oral antibiotic therapy predisposes to the condition which can be treated with topical nystatin or an imidazole cream but any oral candidiasis will also require treatment.

Other napkin area eruptions

These include perianal dermatitis and atopic dermatitis which are common and psoriasis which is rare in the infant.

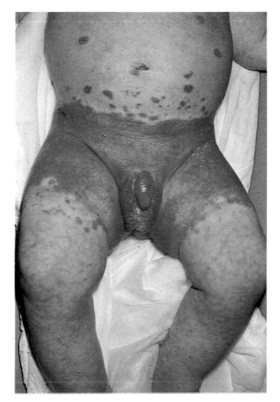

Figure 5.8 **Napkin psoriasis.** Note the well-defined napkin area eruption with psoriasiform spread.

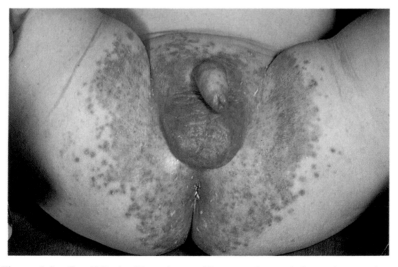

Figure 5.9 **Candidiasis.** Note the satellite pustules and the main eruption.

ERYTHEMATO-SQUAMOUS DISORDERS

Psoriasis

Psoriasis (Figures 5.10–5.17) is a common genetically-determined condition of unknown cause, seen frequently in children. However, onset before the age of 5 years is unusual and before the age of 2 years is rare. In children, the most common type is *guttate psoriasis* which appears abruptly, often after a streptococcal tonsillitis or other infection. The small papular lesions have overlying silvery scales. The guttate eruption persists for up to 3–4 months and resolves spontaneously. However, it is usual for psoriasis of some type to recur within the following 3–5 years.

The *Köbner phenomenon* in which lesions appear along the site of injury may be seen in active psoriasis. However, it is also found in

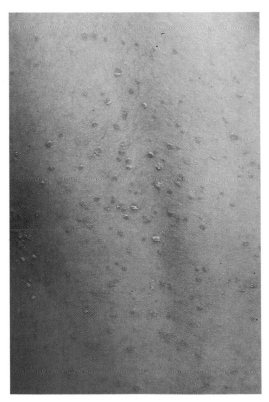

Figure 5.10 **Psoriasis.** Guttate psoriasis in a boy of 5½ years. Close-up of back.

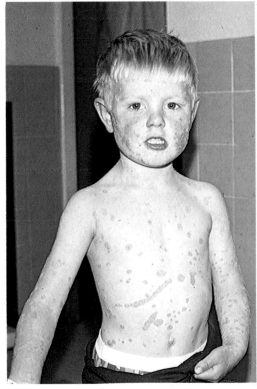

Figure 5.11 **Psoriasis.** Boy of 5 years showing both guttate and larger lesions and Köbner phenomenon. He also has facial involvement.

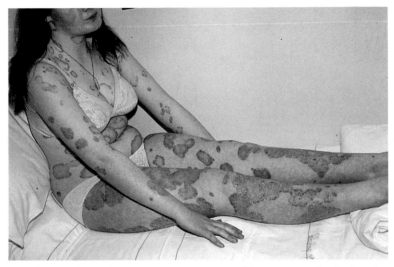

Figure 5.12 **Psoriasis.** Widespread plaque type with many annular lesions in a girl of 16 years.

other conditions such as lichen planus, viral warts and molluscum contagiosum.

The plaque type of psoriasis (*psoriasis vulgaris*) is less common in children and apart from plaques, annular patches of varying sizes may occur. Psoriatic plaques may be encircled by a clear pale zone, the ring of Woronoff.

Patchy thick scaling areas are typical of scalp psoriasis and when scales are removed some hair may be lost but almost always regrows. *Pityriasis amiantacea* describes a condition in which scalp patches occur showing white asbestos-like scales which cling firmly to the hair shafts as they emerge from the scalp and extend some distance along them; in children it is often psoriatic.

Nail changes are seen particularly in chronic psoriasis and are uncommon in children, but onycholysis and pitting may be seen and occasionally nail changes are seen with minimal skin involvement.

Pustular psoriasis is rare in children but it should be mentioned as a warning against the increasing use of topical corticosteroids in the treatment of ordinary psoriasis because their use may precipitate the pustular form. However, in children psoriasis may present as a *pustular acrodermatitis* involving one or two fingers which may co-exist with or be followed later by typical psoriasis elsewhere.

Bland ointments are recommended for guttate psoriasis. Coal tar preparations are useful for psoriasis vulgaris and scalp psoriasis. Coal

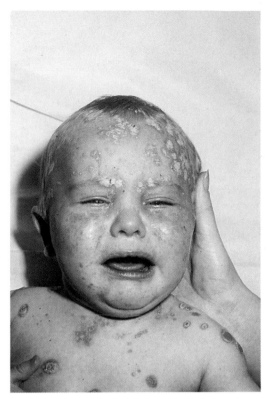

Figure 5.13   **Psoriasis** showing typical scaled psoriatic lesions in an 8-month-old boy; the onset was at the very early age of 7 weeks.

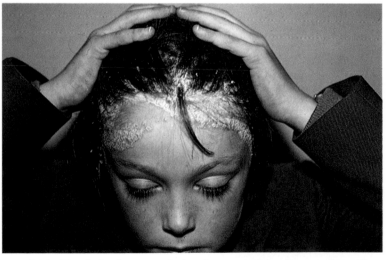

Figure 5.14   **Psoriasis.** Severe scalp involvement with adjacent skin affected.

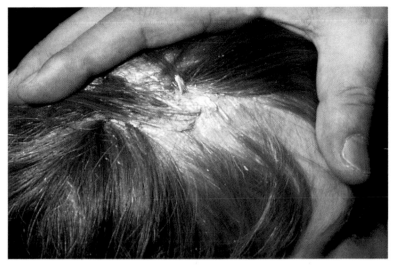

Figure 5.15 **Psoriasis—pityriasis amiantacea** is shown here with thick white scales enveloping hair as it emerges from the scalp. Psoriasis was the underlying disorder in this child.

tar solution can be added to the bath and dithranol (anthralin) is very effective in resistant plaque type of psoriasis. Sunlight and ultraviolet B light (UVB) have a beneficial effect in chronic psoriasis in most individuals; however they are contraindicated in acute guttate or other

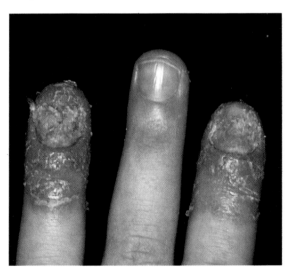

Figure 5.16 **Psoriasis.** This 7½-year-old girl shows pustular acrodermatitis involving two fingers only.

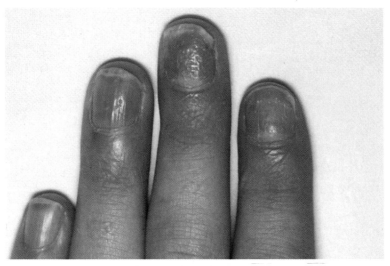

Figure 5.17   **Psoriasis** of nails in same girl as in Figure 5.16 20 months later showing pitting and onycholysis. It is interesting that the middle finger which was unaffected by acrodermatitis shows the most marked pitting.

acute psoriasis and sunburn can induce a Köbner phenomenon. Photochemotherapy (psoralens plus UVA) is not indicated in routine management of childhood psoriasis.

Pityriasis rubra pilaris

This is a rare condition of unknown cause, without specific treatment. The disorder may present in different ways, including a widespread psoriasiform eruption, in which small areas of normal-appearing skin are visible, or with marked palmo-plantar hyperkeratosis showing orange-red discoloration. Localized patches over knees will show follicular papules with hyperkeratotic plugs, giving a rough feel. Many cases will persist for months or even years, but frequently spontaneous remission does occur.

Pityriasis rosea

This condition (Figures 5.18 and 5.19) is a presumed but unproven virus infection of 4–6 weeks duration, most commonly affecting children and young adults. The first lesion is termed the *herald patch* and precedes others by a few days; the rash is typically irritant after a bath. Superficial scaly patches with increased scaling from the centre appear, particularly on the trunk, sometimes noticeably in the line

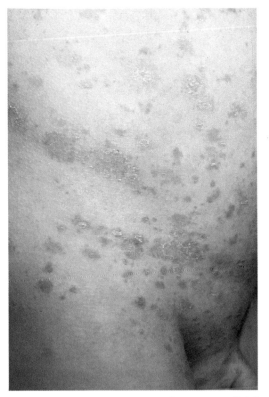 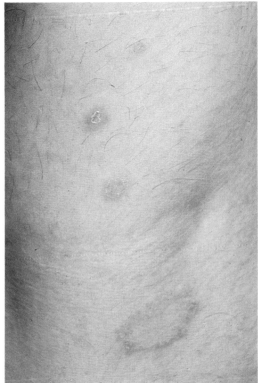

Figure 5.18 **Pityriasis rosea.** Discrete superficial scaling lesions with some showing typical central peeling.

Figure 5.19 **Pityriasis rosea.** Close-up to show scaling lesions behind knee.

of the ribs over the posterior rib cage. Occasionally in acute cases, lesions may be papular or even vesicular at first but some more typical scaling lesions can usually be found sooner or later. Purpuric lesions occur occasionally, but once again more typical lesions peeling at their central portion will also be visible. Maximum incidence is in the months November to February. If irritation is marked, mild or moderately potent topical corticosteroid creams are useful.

Pityriasis lichenoides

This is an uncommon self-limiting vasculitis of unknown cause (Figures 5.20 and 5.21). The basic lesion is a reddish-brown papule and lesions are most marked over trunk and limbs. Different lesions may occur with some haemorrhagic, some necrotic and others showing a removable central scale. There is no systemic upset and any

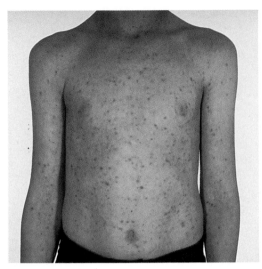

Figure 5.20 **Pityriasis lichenoides.** Widespread haemorrhagic-looking papular eruption over trunk.

itching is usually minimal. If there was such a disorder as chronic varicella this would be its appearance! The course of the condition is variable lasting months to years. Exposure to ultraviolet B light or sunshine may hasten resolution.

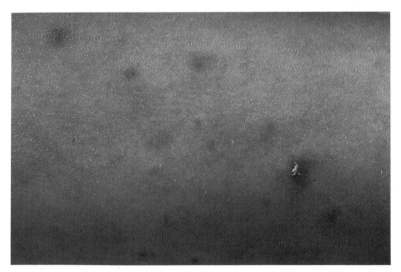

Figure 5.21 **Pityriasis lichenoides.** Close-up of lesions in same boy, one showing a typical mica scale.

Lichen planus

This is a condition of unknown cause rare in children, in which flat-topped violaceous papules appear, typically over fronts of wrists and trunk. There may be mouth and nail involvement.

Lichen nitidus

This condition, although an uncommon self-limiting disorder is particularly seen in children and can be considered a variant of lichen planus. It shows histological features identical to lichen planus yet more focal in nature. Small non-irritant flat-topped papules occur in groups usually over the trunk.

Acropustulosis of infancy

This is a condition (Figure 5.22) that seems to be more common in black infants. It occurs between the ages of 2–10 months. Crops of pruritic erythematous papules become vesico-pustular and appear particularly over palms and soles, but sometimes over the scalp also, a crop appearing over a week or so; then the lesions subside, only to recur a few weeks later.

Antihistamines are helpful in reducing pruritus and the condition resolves spontaneously in the first 2–3 years of life. Before diagnosing the condition the much more common scabies must be excluded.

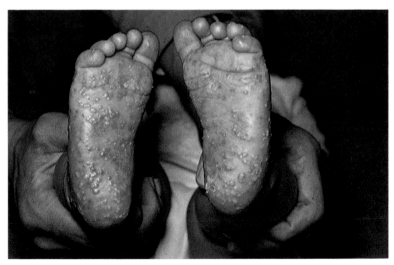

Figure 5.22 **Acropustulosis of infancy.** Pustules over sole in a 5-month-old boy. His mother was of West Indian origin.

REFERENCES

1. Podmore, P., Burrows, D., Eedy, D. J. and Stanford, C. F. (1986). Seborrhoeic eczema—a disease entity or a clinical variant of atopic eczema? *Br. J. Dermatol.,* **115**, 341–50
2. Ilchyshyn, A., Mendelsohn, S. S., Macfarlane, A. and Verbov, J. (1987). *Candida albicans* and infantile seborrhoeic dermatitis. *Br. J. Clin. Pract.,* **41**, 557–9

6

Hair and Nails

CONTENTS

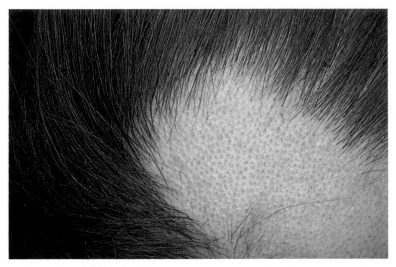

Figure 6.1 **Alopecia areata.** Close-up of an area of alopecia showing exclamation mark hairs between 9 and 2 o'clock.

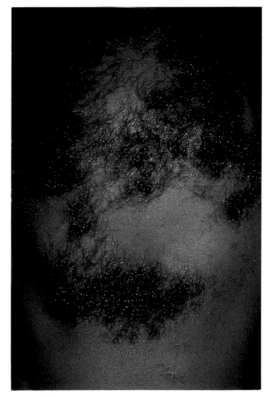

Figure 6.2 **Alopecia areata.** Extensive loss of posterior scalp hair.

HAIR

Hair Loss

Alopecia areata This is the most common form of hair loss in children and a cause of much distress to both children and parents (Figures 6.1–6.3). Hairless smooth areas of skin, usually over the scalp, are visible; remnants of broken-off hairs, visible as exclamation marks, may be seen at the edge of active patches. Early patches in children particularly, may show an irregular outline. The prognosis is good when there are few patches of hair loss, and both parents and patients should be told this with likely regrowth in a 6–12 months, but the more extensive the loss the more guarded should be the prognosis. When associated with atopy the prognosis also tends to be poor. The condition is sometimes recurrent. It has been well discussed in a recent symposium[1].

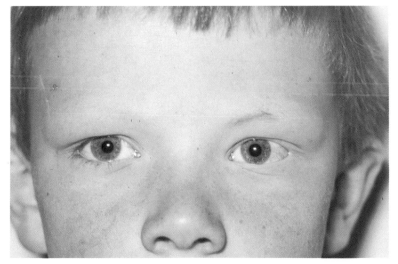

Figure 6.3 **Alopecia areata.** (Left) eyelashes and (right) eyebrow hair were completely lost in this boy.

Traumatic hair loss Traumatic hair loss that is self-inflicted may be intentional or accidental. Thus, pony tails, various ethnic hair styles (Figure 6.4), trendy styles, tight rollers, and hot combs may cause patchy alopecia unintentionally. Head pressure and movement combine to produce the common temporary occipital hair loss seen in infants (Figure 6.5). *Trichotillomania* (Figures 6.6 and 6.7) is the

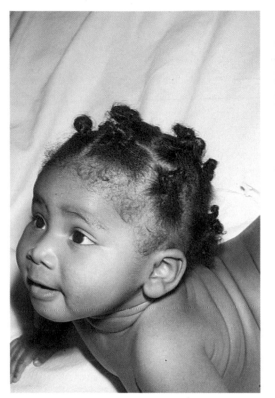

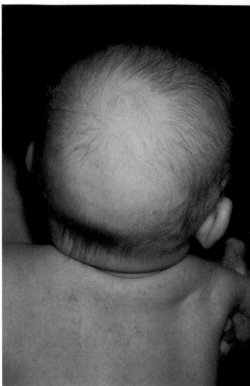

Figure 6.4 **Traumatic hair loss.** Traction alopecia in a 7-month-old Jamaican infant.

Figure 6.5 **Traumatic hair loss.** Occipital hair loss due to head pressure, movement and delayed telogen in a 4-month-old infant.

term sometimes used to describe the self-limiting form of alopecia produced either consciously, or involuntarily as the result of habit. Thus, children may cause breakage of hairs by the common habit of twisting groups of hairs, or they can pull out, or, rarely, cut their own hair intentionally. Usually of no consequence, it can be important if persistent and extensive, posing a major threat, to both child and family in terms of emotional stability; emotional deprivation in the maternal relationship may set off the habit. Clinically, differentiation from alopecia areata is usually based on the irregular outline, bizarre appearance and the presence of short stub-like hairs in trichotillomania. Sometimes scalp hair fall in children may result from others pulling out the hair.

Hair loss due to scalp ringworm is mentioned in Chapter 4.

Hereditary diffuse hair loss   When occurring by itself, it is usually an autosomal dominant trait, and eyebrows and eyelashes may be

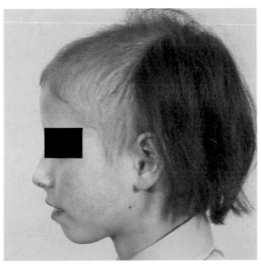

Figure 6.7 **Traumatic hair loss: tricho-tillomania.** Same child as in Figure 6.6 in profile.

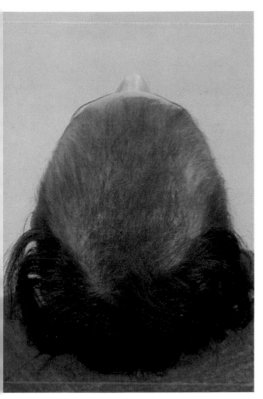

Figure 6.6 **Traumatic hair loss: trichotillo-mania.** Bizarre widespread hair loss in a 9-year-old girl with hair of normal appearance persisting over sides and posterior scalp. All her traumatized hair regrew.

affected as well as the scalp. It is usually permanent. However, hypotrichosis is more commonly just one component in many genodermatoses such as anhidrotic and hidrotic ectodermal dysplasias, Rothmund–Thomson syndrome, focal dermal hypoplasia and acrodermatitis enteropathica.

Scarring alopecia This is the end result of many inflammatory processes resulting in irreversible scarring of the affected area (Figure 6.8). Local infections, trauma and various dermatoses may produce scarring.

Aplasia cutis is a rare developmental deformity, in some cases genetically determined, most commonly affecting the scalp: A crust or ulcer present at birth heals leaving a scar.

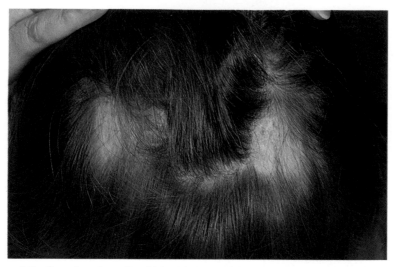

Figure 6.8   Scarring alopecia. Girl of 9 years with two patches of scarring alopecia over the anterior half of scalp. The mother was uncertain whether they were present at birth, but aplasia cutis is likely.

Hair shaft deformities

Monilethrix (beading of hair)   This is an autosomal dominant permanent condition which affects scalp hairs producing partial alopecia but other hairs can be affected. Individual hairs show beading with the elliptical nodes 0.7–1.0 mm apart separated by narrow internodes at which the medulla is lacking. The internodes break transversely so that hair fails to grow to any appreciable length.

Pili torti (twisting of hair)   This indicates multiple 180° twists each no more than a fraction of a millimetre long occurring with scalp hair particularly. It can occur alone as an isolated autosomal dominant condition but may occur in other inherited syndromes. When light is shone on twisted hair at varying angles, a flecking or spangling effect is seen.

Trichorrhexis nodosa   This is a condition in which there is an inherent weakness of the hair shaft so that, with minor trauma such as brushing or shampooing, the shaft readily fractures through the centre of a node.

Woolly hair   This may occur as a localized hair naevus, which is a developmental abnormality, or as an inherited condition in Caucasians affecting the whole scalp and giving the appearance of negroid hair. The latter condition is termed the *woolly hair syndrome* and although usually autosomal dominant it may be autosomal recessive. The onset is at birth with maximum severity in childhood when the curl diameter is approximately 0.5 cm and it is very difficult to brush or comb the woolly wiry hair. A 180° axial rotation of the hair shaft is invariable and trichorrhexis nodosa is common.

Uncombable hair syndrome This syndrome (Figure 6.9) is usually first noticed at around the age of 3 years but may occur earlier or later. The scalp hair is disorderly and remains so despite brushing and combing. On histological examination, hair shafts are seen to show a longitudinal depression and may be triangular. Spontaneous improvement tends to occur. This condition is discussed and many other hair shaft abnormalities in a useful paper by Whiting[2].

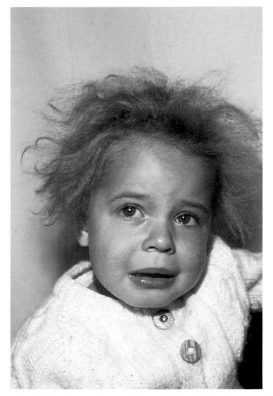

Figure 6.9 **Uncombable hair syndrome.** Since birth this 2½-year-old girl had unruly hair. She slowly improved.

NAILS

Ringworm of the nails is considered in Chapter 4 and psoriatic nails in Chapter 5.

Infections

Apart from ringworm, other infections involving the nails include chronic paronychia and blistering distal dactylitis.

Chronic paronychia   This is seen most commonly in thumb or finger suckers or biters (Figure 6.10). A mixed flora of bacteria and *Candida albicans* is often found. The skin is usually erythematous and glistens. Deformity of the nail is a common complication. Cure requires correction of the sucking habit and treatment of the infection.

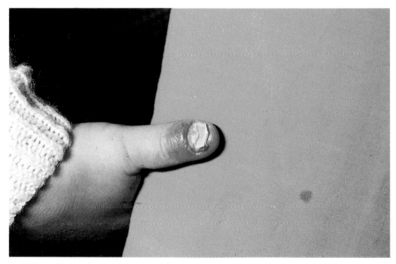

Figure 6.10   **Chronic paronychia.** Illustrated are the inflamed posterior nail-fold and dystrophic nail in this thumb sucker.

Blistering distal dactylitis   This uncommon β-haemolytic streptococcal infection presents as a tender single blister with surrounding erythema over the flexor aspect of a fingertip. The lesion may require incision in addition to oral antibiotic therapy.

Ingrowing toenail

This is not uncommon in childhood (Figure 6.11). In infants a combination of walking and ill-fitting footwear pressure may induce pain, bacterial paronychia and overgrowth of granulation tissue around the

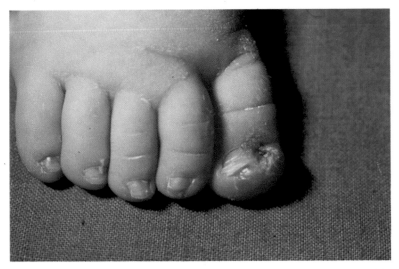

Figure 6.11 **Ingrowing toenail.** The medial nail-fold is inflamed here around the nail plate.

soft pliable nail plate. In addition, incorrect cutting of the toenails is an important factor. However, a primary factor in infants can be unduly prominent skin at the extreme tip of the big toe forming an anterior nail fold which encourages ingrowing and prevents the free end of the big toenail growing normally: This condition may sometimes be genetically determined. For ingrowing toenail, local antiseptic measures will be required and advice to parents regarding avoidance of pressure trauma on the toes. Because of the likelihood of recurrence, surgery should usually be avoided and moreover where there is a prominent anterior nail-fold, this may spontaneously cease to overhang with time allowing normal nail growth.

Malalignment of the big toenail

Ingrowing will also be encouraged by malalignment of the big toenail (Figure 6.12). If lateral deviation of the nail plate is present (i.e. malalignment) and is marked, surgical correction with re-alignment of the whole nail apparatus may be indicated and should be done before the age of 2 years[3]: spontaneous resolution can also occur.

Twenty-nail dystrophy

This is an acquired dystrophy (Figure 6.13), eventually of all 20 nails, that begins in childhood. It is usually of unknown cause, but alopecia

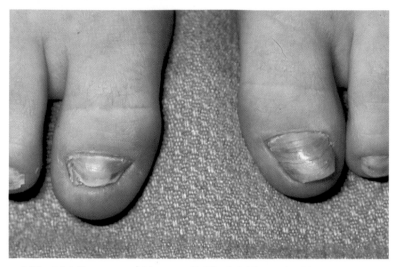

Figure 6.12 **Malalignment of big toenail.** The left big toe in this 8-year-old girl had been deviated laterally since the age of 1 year.

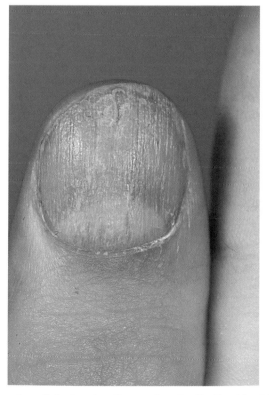

Figure 6.13 **Twenty-nail dystrophy.** Opaque longitudinally-ridged thumb nail with transverse splitting of the free end into layers.

areata or lichen planus are causes. Excessive longitudinal ridging, opacity, and shininess or roughness occur. It tends to be self-limiting and reversible although any nail damage including atrophy or pterygium formation will remain.

Beau's Lines

These are transverse linear depressions of the nails which develop as a reaction to any severe illness or shock that temporarily interrupts nail formation (Figure 6.14). They become visible on the nail plate a few months after the onset of the disease that caused the condition. Since the lines originate under the proximal nail-fold, the date of the illness can be estimated by the distance of the depression from the cuticle.

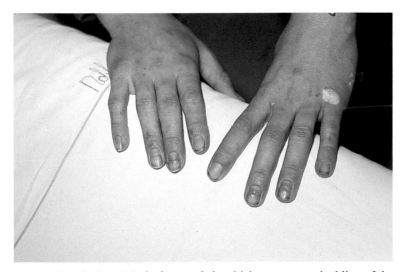

Figure 6.14 **Beau's lines.** Marked example in which temporary shedding of the nails occurred. The boy had had infectious mononucleosis months previously.

Koilonychia

This is seen frequently as a normal finding in the first few months of life due to the thin and soft nail plate. However, a dominant inherited persistent form exists and iron deficiency anaemia is a further cause of flat or spoon-shaped nails.

REFERENCES

1. Thiers, B. H., Bergfeld, W. F., Fiedler-Weiss, V. C., Weston, W. L., Lane, A. T., Price, V. H., Verbov, J. L. and Galen, W. K. (1987). Alopecia Areata Symposium. *Pediatr. Dermatol.,* **4**, 136–58
2. Whiting, D. A. (1987). Structural abnormalities of the hair shaft. *J. Am. Acad. Dermatol.,* **16**, 1–25
3. Baran, R. and Bureau, H. (1983). Congenital malalignment of the big toe-nail as a cause of ingrowing toe-nail in infancy. Pathology and treatment (a study of thirty cases). *Clin. Exp. Dermatol.,* **8**, 619–23

7

Naevi and Nodules

CONTENTS

Subungual exostosis
Recurring digital fibroma
Histiocytosis-X (Langerhans-cell histiocytosis)
    Letterer–Siwe disease

NAEVI

Pigmented naevi

Melanocytic naevus (naevocellular naevus)   These lesions (Figures 7.1–7.4) composed of naevus cells, are divided into intradermal, junctional and compound, depending on the location of the naevus cells. Such naevi are very common, but the majority appear in childhood and adolescence. Face, neck and back are the usual sites and only a very small fraction of the total become malignant, usually in adult life.

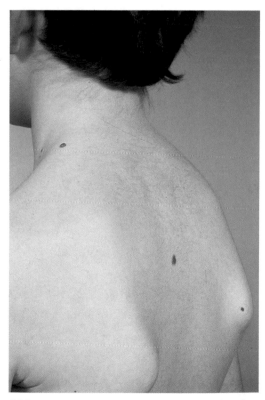

Figure 7.1   **Melanocytic naevus.** Child of 11 years showing three naevi.

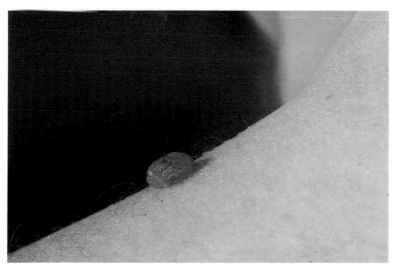

Figure 7.2 **Melanocytic naevus.** Close-up of same child as in Figure 7.1 showing dome-shaped sessile intradermal naevus over neck.

According to a recent study[1] most small congenital naevocellular naevi are speckled at their borders and show increased skin markings when compared with the uninvolved surrounding skin.

Dysplastic naevus These lesions, which are sometimes familial, have an irregular border and are usually larger (5–15 mm or more) and

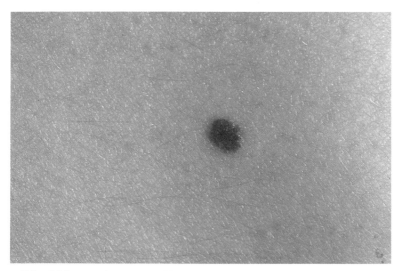

Figure 7.3 **Melanocytic naevus.** Close-up of same child as in Figures 7.1 and 7.2 showing dark-brown macular hairless junctional naevus over right scapula.

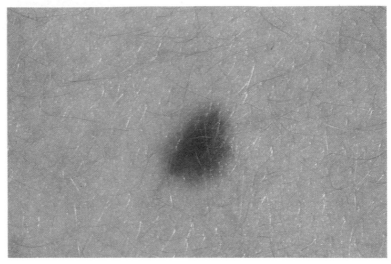

Figure 7.4 **Melanocytic naevus.** Close-up of same child as in Figures 7.1–7.3 showing interscapular slightly raised hairy compound naevus. It is likely to have developed from a purely junctional naevus.

more profuse than acquired ordinary melanocytic naevi. They tend to be multi-coloured, and may have a palpable centre. Such naevi appear as early as 5 or 6 years of age but increase in size and number after puberty. Their importance is that they may be a precursor or marker for malignant melanoma and thus indicate careful and regular observation[2].

Halo naevus (Sutton's naevus)   This is a common single or multiple lesion which presents usually over the trunk with a patch of depigmentation around a central, commonly compound melanocytic naevus (Figure 7.5). The cause of the spontaneous depigmentation is unknown but there is an increased incidence of vitiligo in those with halo naevi. Lesions (halo and central) have a tendency to spontaneous resolution but this may take years.

Spindle-cell naevus (juvenile melanoma)   This presents as a firm smooth-surfaced dome-shaped nodule, usually reddish brown, correlated with the vascularity of the tumour, but it may be black and can have a warty appearance (Figure 7.6). Cells in the lesion are generally spindle-shaped and multinucleated giant cells and mitotic figures are also present. The spindle and giant cells are two features distinguishing the lesion from malignant melanoma.

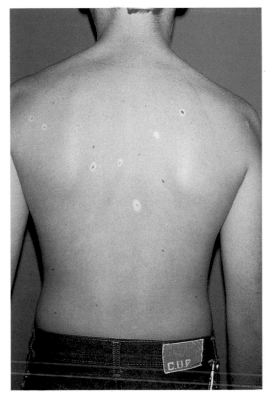

Figure 7.5 **Halo naevus.** Multiple naevi over back.

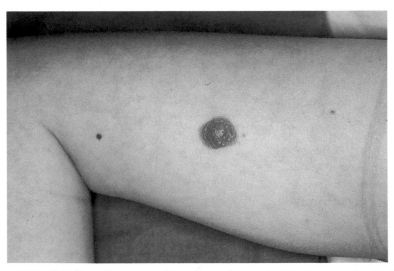

Figure 7.6 **Spindle-cell naevus (juvenile melanoma).** Rather vascular-looking orange-brown nodule over thigh.

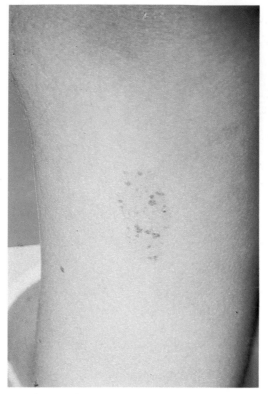

Figure 7.7   **Naevus spilus.** Lesion over upper arm showing dots of darker pigmentation both at the edge and within the patch of pigmentation.

Naevus spilus   This is a solitary brown macule dotted with small brownish-black areas of pigmentation (Figure 7.7). It may be 1 cm or more in diameter and the histology is that of a dermal or junctional melanocytic naevus.

Blue naevus   This presents as a rounded area of blue or blue-black dermal pigmentation usually slightly raised and smooth surfaced, produced by aberrant collections of functioning melanocytes. Common sites are dorsa of hands and fcet, buttocks and face. Lesions may appear at birth or at any age. There are two types: the ordinary, and the less frequently seen cellular blue naevus which tends to be larger than 1 cm in diameter, and which shows islands of large cells on histology not present in the ordinary blue naevus.

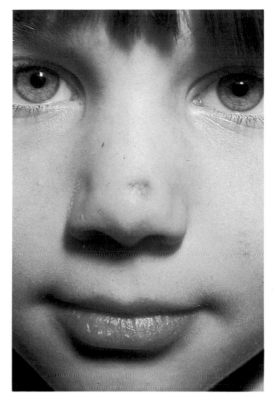

Figure 7.8 **Spider naevus.** The lesion is visible over nose.

Dermal naevi

Spider telangiectasis (spider naevus) This consists of a central arteriole with radiating vessels (Figure 7.8). Such lesions are common and occur on the upper half of the body. Lesions occurring in healthy children tend to persist indefinitely. The central vessel can be destroyed with cautery or diathermy without any anaesthetic in the older child.

Angioma serpiginosum This is a rare disorder of upper dermal capillaries and venules which show localized dilatations[3] and it occurs mainly in females. Onset is usually in childhood rather than infancy, and lower limbs and buttocks are the preferred sites. It begins as one or more red or purple puncta which extend over a period of months or years. Lesions commonly follow the livedo patterning of the skin and there may be a background of diffuse erythema. Individual puncta may disappear and complete resolution may occur but is uncommon.

Lymphangioma circumscriptum   This is the most common form of lymphangioma and presents at birth or in early childhood. It is characterized by groups of deep-seated thick-walled vesicles that resemble frog spawn. Frequently there is an haemangiomatous component. Although referred to as 'circumscriptum' larger lesions particularly, may reveal a more widespread abnormality on investigation and this is very relevant if any surgical treatment is contemplated. Common sites include proximal limbs, chest wall and perineum.

Juvenile xanthogranuloma   This is a self-limiting asymptomatic condition (Figure 7.9) seen in infants and young children, more common in whites than in negroes. Single or multiple yellow, brown or reddish papules occur. Histopathology reveals typical Touton giant cells which are histiocytes loaded with lipid. There is no evidence of abnormal lipid metabolism elsewhere and the lesions nearly always disappear before puberty.

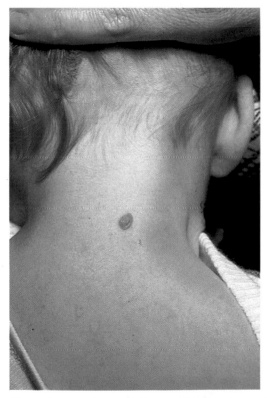

Figure 7.9   **Juvenile xanthogranuloma.** Solitary soft yellow-brown lesion over back of neck.

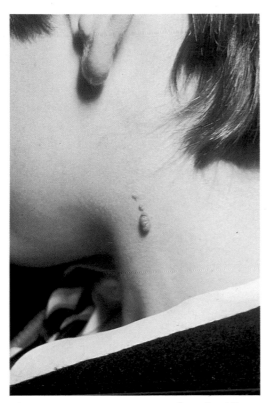

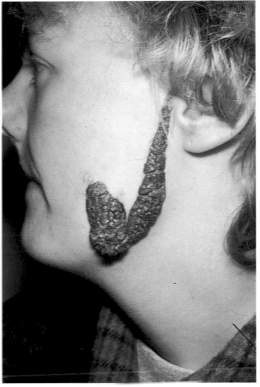

Figure 7.10 **Verrucous naevus.** Localized linear lesions over side of neck.

Figure 7.11 **Verrucous naevus.** Well-defined striking 'tick' lesion over face. She had reached the age of 19 years before plucking up courage to attend the clinic. It was excised by a plastic surgeon with an excellent result.

Epidermal naevi

Verrucous

Localized These lesions are usually solitary presenting at birth or appearing in infancy or early childhood and growing with the individual (Figure 7.10 and 7.11). They are skin-coloured or brown, raised with a rough warty surface. They vary in size and tend to be linear when over limbs. Histopathology shows hyperkeratosis, papillomatosis, and acanthosis. If requiring treatment, excision is recommended; cryotherapy or cautery will be followed by recurrence sooner or later.

Widespread In this, naevus lesions are extensive and may form wavy transverse bands on the trunk and longitudinal often spiral streaks on

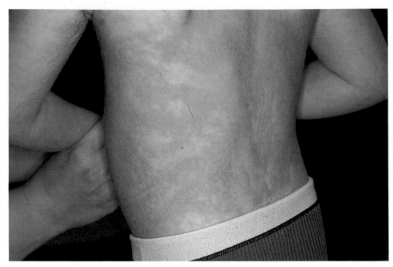

Figure 7.12 **Verrucous naevus.** Widespread naevus in a boy of 2½ years which became more warty and widespread as he grew older.

the limbs (Figure 7.12). Some of these naevi show histological features of epidermolytic hyperkeratosis (see Chapter 2) and in some cases may be a manifestation of that disorder. Extensive unilateral verrucous naevi are sometimes referred to as *naevus unius lateris.* Verrucous naevi usually of the widespread type, may uncommonly be associated with developmental defects in other systems and such cases are referred to as the *epidermal naevus syndrome.*

Inflamed linear epidermal naevus This usually appears in infancy and is four times more common in females (Figure 7.13). It is pruritic and consists of scaly patches which appear as a linear eruption looking eczematous or psoriasiform; it may appear warty. Most occur unilaterally over lower limbs and buttocks and may be very extensive. Histopathology reveals hyperkeratosis, parakeratosis, spongiosis and a dermal inflammatory infiltrate.

Sebaceous naevus This is an uncommon but important congenital lesion containing both epidermal and dermal elements (Figure 7.14). Most common over the scalp and usually single, they appear here as smooth, slightly raised, hairless waxy plaques, yellow orange in colour and linear or somewhat oval in shape. It becomes thickened and more raised during late childhood and adolescence. Histologically there is an increase in the number of sebaceous glands which may also be

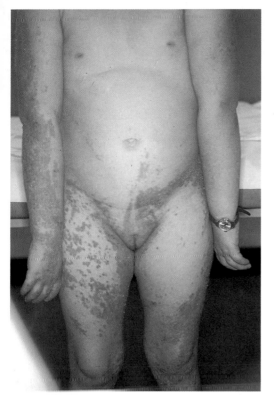

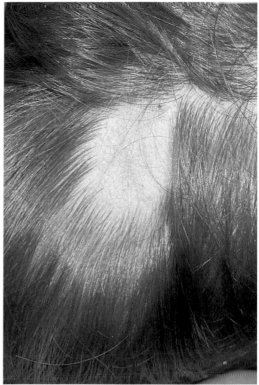

Figure 7.13 **Inflamed linear epidermal naevus.** Girl of 5 years with irritant psoriasiform eruption (courtesy of Dr. T. W. Stewart).

Figure 7.14 **Sebaceous naevus.** A 3½-year-old child with this slightly raised somewhat orange-looking warty hairless scalp patch.

enlarged and associated with hypertrophy and hyperkeratosis of the epidermis. Benign or malignant transformation, particularly basal cell carcinoma, is not uncommon in these lesions and usually occurs from the fourth decade. Excision should be carried out in adolescence or early adult life as a precaution.

Naevoid hypertrichosis The abnormal presence of excess hair may occur as a developmental defect in the absence of any other abnormality (Figure 7.15).

Faun-tail naevus Sometimes an abnormal growth of hair (a faun-tail) or other skin lesion over the midline of the spine, usually in the sacral region, may indicate spina bifida (Figure 7.16). In view of the possible association of spinal cord abnormalities with spina

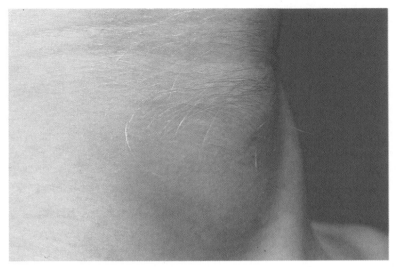

Figure 7.15   **Naevoid hypertrichosis.** A girl of 5 years with excess hair present since 7 months old; localized to front of neck. Treated by cutting at intervals.

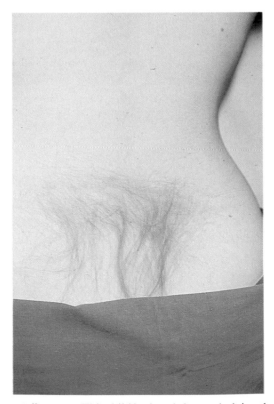

Figure 7.16   **Faun-tail naevus.** This child had no defect underlying the hypertrichosis.

bifida which may not produce symptoms until late childhood, the presence of any such skin lesions should lead to full neurological examination.

Some other pigmented and vascular dermal naevi have been mentioned in Chapter 2.

NODULES

Granuloma telangiectaticum (pyogenic granuloma)

This is a vascular nodule which develops rapidly often at the site of a recent injury particularly over a finger. It is usually a dull-red fleshy polypoid lesion which may be pedunculated and easily bleeds with trauma (Figure 7.17). The treatment is curettage, followed by diathermy coagulation of the base. Lesions may recur with initial treatment and a few may require excision.

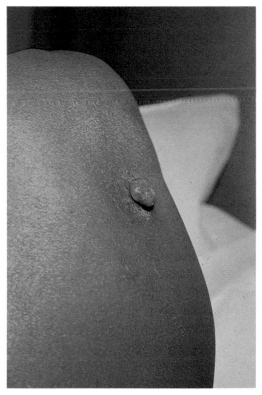

Figure 7.17 **Pyogenic granuloma.** Girl of 10 years with lesion over scapular region.

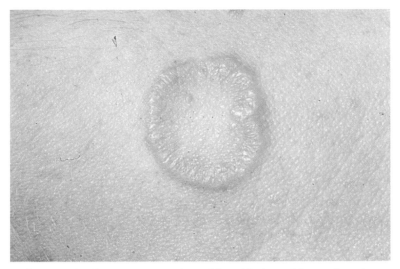

Figure 7.18 **Granuloma annulare.** Ringed lesion with papular edge.

Granuloma annulare

This may occur anywhere but is usually over bony prominences and especially over hands and feet (Figure 7.18). Children and young adults are most commonly affected and incidence is higher in females. Early lesions begin as smooth flesh-coloured papules that slowly undergo central involution and peripheral extension to form oval or irregular rings with elevated often beaded borders. Lesions may be single or multiple and are usually 1–3 cm in diameter but more extensive patches, sometimes with a somewhat violaceous hue, may occur. Deeper subcutaneous lesions are also seen. Lesions tend to disappear spontaneously and attempts at treatment are unrewarding.

Necrobiosis lipoidica

This is a degenerative disorder of dermal connective tissue seen particularly in diabetics (Figure 7.19); it may also precede the onset of diabetes by a few years. The disorder may occur at any age. Lesions are most common over the pretibial areas and they begin as an erythematous papule or patch which gradually enlarges and develops slowly into a brownish-yellow sclerotic plaque. The centre of the plaque is often atrophic with a translucent surface. Treatment of the lesions is unsatisfactory and they are often best left untreated. Early lesions can sometimes be aborted with intralesional triamcinolone although this may produce ulceration in older lesions.

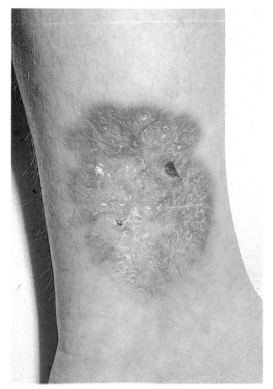

Figure 7.19 **Necrobiosis lipoidica.** Close-up of leg lesion in a diabetic girl of 15 years with outer portion showing telangiectasia, and yellowish colour probably due to carotene. Two years before this photograph was taken, the central portion of the necrobiotic patch had ulcerated and the ulcerated area was excised and a skin graft applied.

Subungual exostosis

This is a solitary fibrous nodule on the terminal border of the distal phalanx of a toe or finger, particularly the big toe. Lesions may be due to trauma or occur spontaneously. They are not usually seen under the age of 4 years. A small flesh-coloured growth develops beneath, and projects sharply beyond the free edge of the nail often detaching it. It is often painful as it grows. Treatment of choice is excision by an orthopaedic surgeon.

Recurring digital fibroma

This presents as a firm shiny dome-shaped nodule or nodules around a finger or toe nail. Lesions tend to involute spontaneously but may take a few years to do so and occasionally surgery may be required in some complicated cases[4].

Histiocytosis-X (Langerhans-cell histiocytosis)

Letterer–Siwe disease, eosinophilic granuloma and Hand–Schüller–Christian disease are rare variants of a single clinico-pathological entity affecting tissue histiocytes. Previously considered a malignant disease it is more likely that it has an immunological basis. Most affected individuals have a deficiency of circulating suppressor (T8) lymphocytes and an increased peripheral blood helper (T4): suppressor (T8) ratio. Spontaneous remission of disease has been associated with return of the T4: T8 ratio to normal. It is accepted that patients with single system disease (usually bone or lymph node) have a good prognosis with a high rate of spontaneous remission and negligible mortality. The management of the child with multisystem disease is controversial but the mortality of such disease has hardly declined since the introduction of chemotherapy[5] and such treatment can itself have harmful side-effects. Immune replacement is emphasized nowadays rather than immune suppression.

Letterer–Siwe disease   The infant presents with a scaly seborrhoeic sometimes purpuric eruption often involving the napkin area but it may be widespread. Scanty sterile pustules over the trunk are another presentation in the infant. Ulceration, particularly of flexures, may occur and ulcers may become infected. Failure to respond to conventional therapy is an important diagnostic point[6]. There may be discharging ears, hepatosplenomegaly, lung and bone involvement and anaemia and thrombocytopenia. Skin biopsy of suspect lesions is essential, demonstrating proliferation of well-differentiated histiocytes.

REFERENCES

1. Alper, J. C. and Holmes, L. B. (1983). The incidence and significance of birthmarks in a cohort of 4641 newborns. *Pediatr. Dermatol.* **1**, 58–68
2. Hoss, D. M. and Grant-Kels, J. M. (1986). Significant melanocytic lesions in infancy, childhood and adolescence. In Hurwitz, S. (ed.) *Dermatologic Clinics. Pediatric Dermatology*, Vol. 4, pp. 29–44 (Philadelphia: W. B. Saunders)
3. Chavaz, P. and Laughier, P. (1981). Angiome serpigineux de Hutchison: Étude ultrastructurale. *Ann. Dermatol. Venereol.*, **108**, 429–36
4. Ryman, W. and Bale, P. (1985). Recurring digital fibromas of infancy. *Aust. J. Dermatol.*, **26**, 113–17
5. Broadbent, V. and Pritchard, J. (1985). Histiocytosis X. Current controversies. *Arch. Dis. Child.*, **60**, 605–7
6. Wong, E., Holden, C. A., Broadbent, V. and Atherton, D. J. (1986). Histiocytosis X presenting as intertrigo and responding to topical nitrogen mustard. *Clin. Exp. Dermatol.*, **11**, 183–7

8

Connective-Tissue Disorders

CONTENTS

SCLERODERMA

Morphoea

This type of scleroderma localized to the skin, occurs in various forms. In the *common form* (Figure 8.1) there is a localized, slowly enlarging plaque, in which the skin is firm and bound down to underlying tissues; there is usually no muscle involvement. Clinically, a non-descript localized red or purplish area appears which then becomes indurated. It is commonly seen on the trunk in the form of an oval-shaped area often with a violaceous zone surrounding it in active lesions. Lesions are single or few in number and tend to resolve spontaneously.

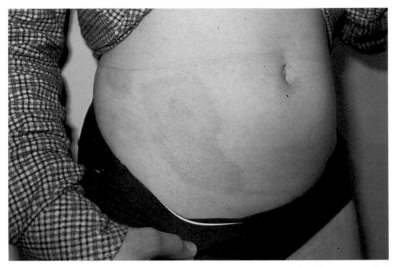

Figure 8.1 **Morphoea.** Large patch over abdomen with small adjacent patch. Note the active edge of the main lesion.

In the *linear form*, which is usually persistent, sclerosis is limited to one area and may or may not be extensive. However, if the scalp is affected, with sclerosis of both skin and underlying structures, there can be progression to a facial hemiatrophy. In a rare linear form of morphoea in children, *disabling pansclerotic morphoea* (Figures 8.2

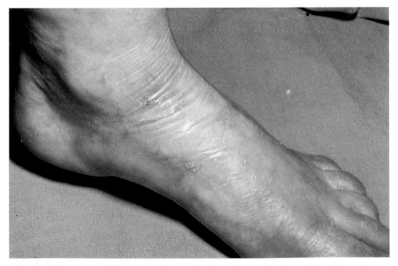

Figure 8.2 **Morphoea.** Here showing binding down of skin of foot in a girl of 5½ years.

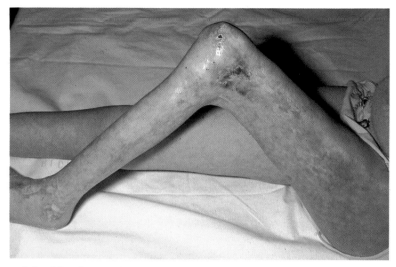

Figure 8.3 **Morphoea.** Four years later the same child as in Figure 8.2 with pansclerotic morphoea had involvement of the whole lower limb with muscle involvement, limb shortening, a stiff ankle and contraction at the knee. She was treated with oral penicillamine with no improvement. A few years later the condition burnt itself out but left a wizened limb.

and 8.3), limb lesions may gradually extend to involve the whole limb with atrophy of underlying muscle and bone, and some degree of arrest of growth is likely: If extensive over a lower limb, shortening and limp are inevitable and amputation due to impaired circulation may, rarely, be necessary.

Progressive systemic sclerosis

The initial manifestation is commonly Raynaud's syndrome, although weight loss and weakness may also be early symptoms. Visible skin changes begin in the fingers and can remain localized here. The fingers may be swollen initially but then the skin becomes bound down appearing shiny and there may be both hyper- and hypo-pigmentation. Later atrophic changes occur with thinning, telangiectasia, and subcutaneous atrophy. Calcinosis, finger-tip ulceration, and a characteristic facies with beaked nose and puckering of mouth can also occur. Linear telangiectases over the posterior nail-folds are common. It is important to assess pulmonary, bowel and renal function regularly in these patients. The course is unpredictable and spontaneous improvement can occur but renal and cardiac failure are serious complications.

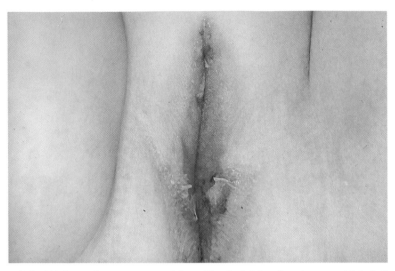

Figure 8.4 **Lichen sclerosus et atrophicus.** Eroded skin of perineum which followed blistering in a 9½-year-old girl. The condition virtually resolved within 3-4 years of onset. This disorder must not be misdiagnosed as sexual abuse.

LICHEN SCLEROSUS ET ATROPHICUS

This is a condition of unknown cause closely allied to morphoea but lesions are usually smaller and in females often involve the vulva (Figure 8.4). It can occur at any age and 90% of cases are females. Well-defined atrophic changes occur in the skin over the clitoris and labia minora and lesions often extend to the perianal region giving a figure-of-eight pattern. Vaginal discharge and pruritus vulvae may be complained of in children and erythema and quite marked blistering may also be seen. The prognosis is usually good with complete resolution. Potent topical corticosteroids have a place when blistering occurs or if pruritus is marked.

LUPUS ERYTHEMATOSUS

In children and adolescents, it is usually of the systemic type and resembles the adult disease clinically and immunologically. Neonatal lupus erythematosus is considered in Chapter 2.

Arthritis, arthralgia, fever and skin eruptions are the most common presenting features. The facial skin eruption may be a widespread erythema with or without oedema, erythema over the butterfly area of the face, or with time, chronic discoid patches. Light-sensitivity occurs in about one-third of patients. More widespread eruptions may also occur. Livedo reticularis, a physical sign with many causes which indicates capillary and venous stasis in cooled skin, may be present and scalp alopecia which is usually diffuse, may be seen. Treatment depends on the degree of systemic involvement and many children will respond simply to bed rest, salicylates and avoidance of sun exposure.

DERMATOMYOSITIS

This is an inflammatory disorder primarily affecting skin and striated muscle but also often involving the gastrointestinal tract. In children, skin signs tend to be florid and muscle pain and tenderness marked: Any association with malignancy is rare. Girls are affected twice as frequently as boys and the mean age of onset in childhood is about 7 years. Muscle weakness involving the proximal limb muscles and anterior neck muscles is the most common first symptom. The skin

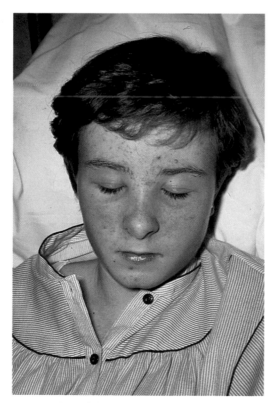

Figure 8.5   **Dermatomyositis.** Violaceous erythema is visible over cheeks and around eyes.

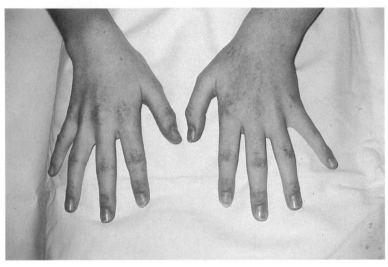

Figure 8.6 **Dermatomyositis**. Same child as in Figure 8.5 showing erythema over posterior nail-folds, proximal interphalangeal joints and knuckles.

eruption consists of violaceous often somewhat oedematous patches that may enlarge and coalesce and thus come to involve fairly extensive areas of skin. The face is most commonly involved especially the periorbital areas and also the upper chest, elbows, knees, knuckles and around the nails (Figures 8.5 and 8.6). Calcinosis develops more commonly in children than in adults and occurs in about half the cases in the healing phase, and the deposits, which are usually subcutaneous and often over joints, have a tendency to ulcerate and discharge. Sometimes calcinosis decreases as the child gets older. The main pathological feature of juvenile dermatomyositis is a vasculitis affecting the small arteries and veins of muscle, skin, subcutaneous tissue and gastrointestinal tract. Prognosis is variable and many children recover completely without any specific therapy but oral corticosteroid therapy preferably in low dosage and short duration[1] has a place in some cases.

POLYARTERITIS NODOSA

This is a rare disease at any age. In the systemic disease which is divided into infantile and childhood groups in children, eruptions tend to be non-specific and include livedo reticularis, erythemas,

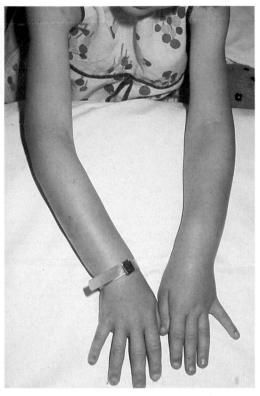

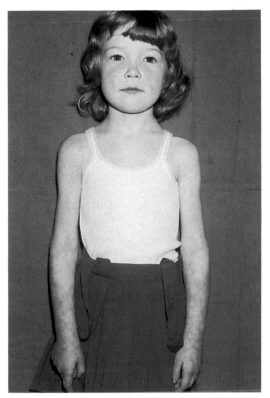

Figure 8.7 **Cutaneous polyarteritis nodosa.** Note the swollen forearms and back of left hand.

Figure 8.8 **Cutaneous polyarteritis nodosa.** Five months later, the girl in Figure 8.7 is much better but livedo reticularis is visible over forearms, hands and cheeks.

urticaria or purpura. *Kawasaki disease* is considered a variant of infantile polyarteritis nodosa. Childhood polyarteritis nodosa is similar to the disease in adults.

In its *benign cutaneous form* (Figures 8.7 and 8.8), polyarteritis nodosa affects the skin only, or it may affect skin, skeletal muscles, and peripheral nerves. Clinically cutaneous polyarteritis nodosa presents as nodules generally on the lower part of the legs. They may be symptomless or extremely painful but they usually resolve spontaneously without scarring, although ulceration can occur. These nodules are associated with livedo reticularis. It is the nodulation rather than the livedo that is the hallmark of the cutaneous disease and these nodules show an arteritic histology typical of polyarteritis nodosa.

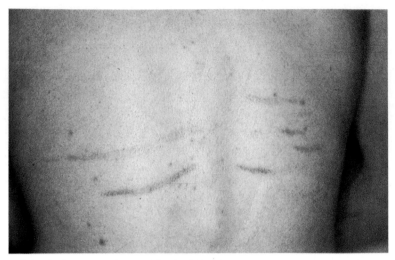

Figure 8.9 **Striae atrophicae.** If looked for they are a common normal finding in older children. Illustrated here are recently-appearing transverse lesions which will flatten later.

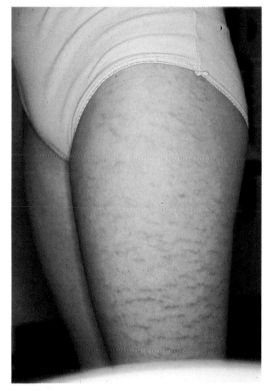

Figure 8.10 **Striae atrophicae.** Here, over thigh in a girl of 12 years.

STRIAE ATROPHICAE

These are a common normal finding at puberty and later (Figures 8.9 and 8.10); their normality is frequently unrecognized. Such striae may first develop soon after the appearance of pubic hair. The commonest sites are the lumbosacral region and outer thighs in boys, and the thighs, buttocks and breasts in girls. At first pink, raised and weal-like, they soon become flat, smooth and bluish in colour. They tend to be linear and these adolescent striae get less noticeable with increasing age. They may occur in thin as well as obese individuals.

KELOID

This represents an exaggerated connective-tissue response to skin injury. Black persons and other darker-skinned individuals are more susceptible and the tendency is often familial. Lesions are pink, smooth, and rubbery and they tend to increase in size long after healing has taken place, proliferating beyond the area of the original wound. Small keloids are relatively common after varicella although they usually follow only one or two of many apparently identical lesions.

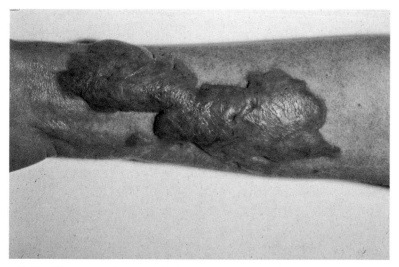

Figure 8.11 **Hypertrophic scar.** The forearm was scalded by steam from a kettle six months previously in this 8-year-old boy. Much spontaneous flattening would be expected within the next few years and there was visible improvement six months after this picture was taken.

HYPERTROPHIC SCARS

These tend to stay within the margin of the lesion (Figure 8.11). Although fresh scars are often hypertrophic, with passage of time and patience, unlike keloids, they contract and become less apparent. It is most important to mention this to parents, following scalds, for instance, for often in children the most unsightly scars will flatten spontaneously within a few years.

REFERENCE

1. Miller, G., Heckmatt, J. Z. and Dubowitz, V. (1983). Drug treatment of juvenile dermatomyositis. *Arch. Dis. Child.*, **58**, 445–50

9

Vascular Disorders and Drug Eruptions

CONTENTS

    Oral corticosteroids
  Local reactions to vaccines
      Bacillus Calmette–Guérin vaccine (BCG)
      Triple vaccine (diphtheria, tetanus, whooping cough)

URTICARIA

Ordinary urticaria

This is sometimes referred to as nettle rash or hives and is a transient itchy erythematous eruption characterized by the appearance of flesh-coloured weals (Figure 9.1). It is due to a local increased permeability of capillaries and small venules. It may be associated with angioedema in which swelling of the lips, eyelids, genitalia, tongue or larynx can occur. Giant urticaria refers to the condition when widespread areas

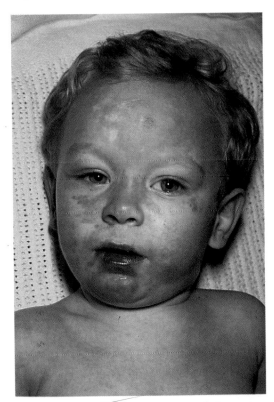

Figure 9.1 **Urticaria.** Affected face is shown but no definite cause was elicited.

of skin are affected. Some residual purpura at lesional sites may occur. Ordinary urticaria as described above is very common and important causes are drugs, food, inhalants, or infections, although many cases are of unknown cause. Acute attacks respond to oral antihistamines and angioedema usually responds also, but if threatening the airway, subcutaneous or intramuscular adrenaline injection 1 in 1000, 0.2–0.5 ml is indicated, and this can be followed if required by intravenous or intramuscular hydrocortisone.

Physical urticarias

Dermographism, cold urticaria, and cholinergic urticaria are the types most frequently seen.

Dermographism (factitious urticaria)   This indicates wealing after the skin is firmly stroked or rubbed (Figure 9.2). It can be observed in at least 5% of normal people, and may or may not be symptomatic.

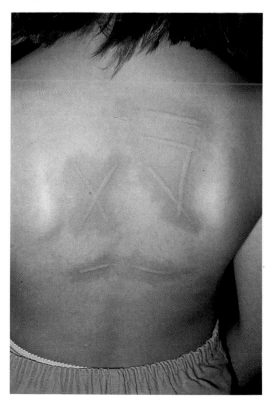

Figure 9.2 **Urticaria.** Here demonstrating **dermographism** in a girl of 10 years.

It may begin in childhood and can give rise to considerable pruritus. The wealing tendency with light trauma persists for months or years.

Cold urticaria   This is usually idiopathic in children and may be inherited or acquired. The inherited form is autosomal dominant and becomes apparent in infancy with urticaria appearing 30 minutes after exposure to cold and lasting up to 48 hours. The acquired form may appear at any age and may be mild or severe. It is important to warn severely affected patients of the possible danger of ice-cream, swimming and bathing because histamine is released and if a large area of skin or mucosa is cooled, this may be hazardous.

Cholinergic urticaria   This is a chronic disorder that may be seen in the older child, characterized by distinctive small 2–3 mm diameter weals or erythema, precipitated by exercise, heat and emotional stress. The acute eruption usually subsides within 30 minutes.

HEREDITARY ANGIOEDEMA

This is a rare autosomal dominant condition due to deficiency of C1 inhibitor. It usually starts in early childhood and presents with subcutaneous swellings often accompanied by abdominal pain. There is no urticaria. The danger in some families is of laryngeal obstruction due to oedema. Infusion of fresh frozen plasma is effective in severe acute attacks and a purified C1 inhibitor preparation is now also available for emergency treatment[1].

ERYTHEMA

Erythema nodosum

This presents with discrete painful red nodules, which may become confluent over the shins (Figure 9.3). Streptococcal infections and, much less likely, primary tuberculous infection, are the most common of many causes; no cause at all is found in about 30% of patients. It is possible that lesions result from the formation or deposition of immune complexes at the site. Lesions less commonly appear over thighs, arms and even over the face. Attacks last 3–6 weeks and the nodules leave bruise-like discoloration as they resolve.

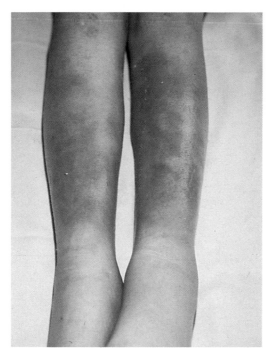

Figure 9.3 **Erythema nodosum.** Painful inflammatory shin nodules, discrete at first but some becoming confluent, in a girl of 11 years. Note associated ankle swelling. E. nodosum must not be mistaken for cellulitis.

Erythema multiforme

This is an inflammatory condition that affects skin and mucous membranes (Figures 9.4 and 9.5). It often occurs without an obvious cause but it has many causes. Herpes simplex and mycoplasma are well-known precipitating causes but drugs are not an important cause in children. Following herpes simplex, erythema multiforme may appear 1–2 weeks later. The target or *iris lesion* is a well-recognised sign and consists of a purple centre surrounded by an erythematous ring; when severe the centre of this target lesion consists of a vesicle or rarely a bulla. Lesions occur over the hands, feet, elbows and knees and there may also be painful ulcers over the buccal mucosa and in more severe cases other mucosae. Attacks usually last for 2–3 weeks but may recur. Target lesions are not always present and an erythematous maculopapular eruption with the characteristic distribution may sometimes occur. The condition is sometimes subdivided into minor and major forms, the most severe bullous form with mucosal involvement being Stevens–Johnson syndrome a major form in which systemic steroids

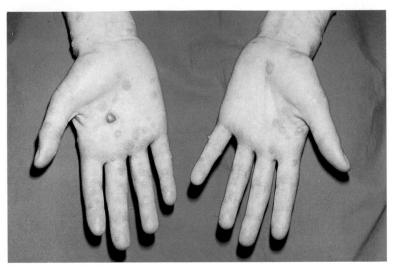

Figure 9.4 **Erythema multiforme.** Typical target lesions with a haemorrhagic blister over right palm.

and antibiotics are required. Systemic and topical acyclovir commenced early in a simplex attack may be useful in preventing erythema multiforme in those with frequent recurrent simplex complicated by erythema multiforme. Mouth washes and oral antihistamines have a place in the routine management of erythema multiforme.

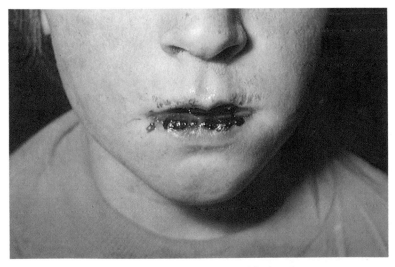

Figure 9.5 **Erythema multiforme.** Lip involvement.

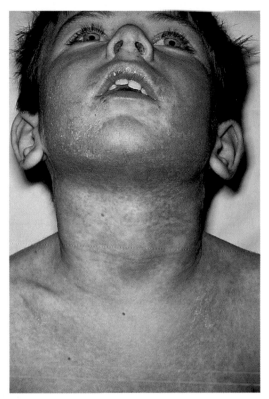

Figure 9.6   **Toxic erythema.** Boy of 8 years with generalized morbilliform eruption followed by peeling. No definite cause was found.

Toxic Erythema

This is a term sometimes used to describe scarlatiniform or morbilliform eruptions (Figure 9.6) due to drugs (see exanthematic drug eruptions, below), virus or bacterial infections or of unknown cause. It is distinct from the transient toxic erythema of the newborn (see Chapter 2). The scarlatiniform eruption consists of diffuse erythema of acute onset or sometimes an identical eruption localized to areas such as palms and soles. Spontaneous resolution usually followed by desquamation occurs in 2–3 weeks. Known causes include the exotoxins of the haemolytic *Streptococcus* and rarely *Staphylococcus* causing scarlet fever, and drugs. Morbilliform eruptions are usually due to virus infections or drugs.

Annular erythema

This term indicates ringed erythematous lesions. We shall consider just two entities, both uncommon but striking in appearance.

Erythema annulare centrifugum (EAC)   This presents as a small pink papule which gradually extends over days or weeks forming an erythematous ring as the central area flattens and fades; the edge is often scaly. Lesions, which may itch slightly, are more often multiple and tend to occur over buttocks, thighs and upper arms. The eruption may come and go over many years and a cause is seldom found.

Erythema chronicum migrans (ECM)   This is a skin reaction to a tick bite. It is recognized as the earliest feature of Lyme disease, an infection caused by the spirochaete *Borrelia burgdorferi* and transmitted via the bite of a tick (*Ixodes ricinus* in Europe and *Ixodes dammini* in the USA). Unlike EAC, lesions are usually solitary and typically begin over exposed areas. The lesion has a slowly advancing indurated border which may extend widely, with central clearing. ECM responds to oral penicillin. In Lyme disease, ECM may be accompanied by constitutional symptoms and is sometimes followed by neurological, cardiac or arthritic symptoms. Diagnosis of Lyme disease is clinical although there may be no bite history, and is confirmed by indirect immunofluorescence or an enzyme-linked immunosorbent assay[2].

PURPURA

Henoch–Schönlein purpura (anaphylactoid purpura)

This is an allergic vasculitis and the most common childhood vasculitis (Figures 9.7 and 9.8). In about one-third of patients the purpura is preceded by an upper respiratory-tract infection. Purpura predominantly over lower limbs and buttocks may be associated with joint pains or with abdominal and renal complications. Lesions may be urticarial initially and in severe cases, purpuric lesions can become necrotic ulcers particularly over the lower legs. Oedema of the face, hands, arms, feet, and scrotum is not uncommon. Arthritis develops in over half the patients, and knees and ankles are most frequently involved. Abdominal symptoms due to vasculitis of gastro-intestinal vessels present most commonly as colic but occult or frank bleeding, intussusception as a result of bleeding, and vomiting may occur. Renal involvement is usually just a transient microscopic haematuria but a

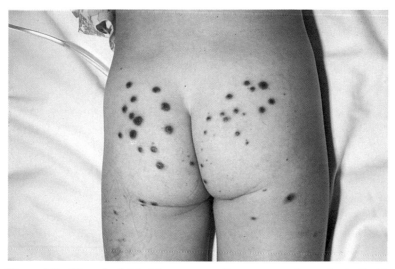

Figure 9.7 **Henoch–Schönlein purpura.** Purpura over buttocks is florid.

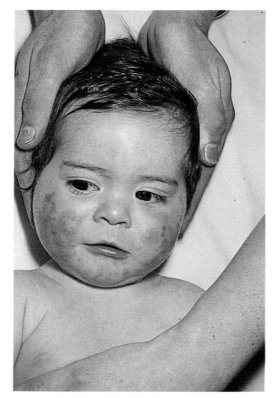

Figure 9.8 **Henoch–Schönlein purpura.** Facial lesions are not uncommon in this disorder.

few patients progress to renal failure. The condition usually settles over a few weeks but can be recurrent. Systemic steroids are unhelpful except in the presence of severe abdominal symptoms.

Idiopathic thrombocytopenic purpura

This tends to be of acute onset and self-limiting in children (Figure 9.9). There are no symptoms other than those due to the effects of bleeding. Bleeding occurs into the skin with petechiae or ecchymoses and may occur in any organ. If treated, corticosteroids or intravenous IgG are used[3].

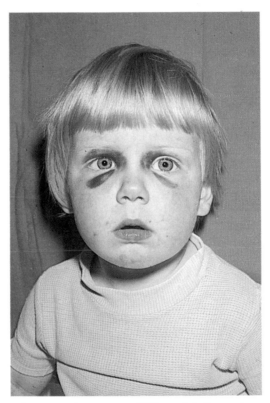

Figure 9.9 **Thrombocytopenic purpura.** Differential diagnosis would include non-accidental injury.

Pigmented purpuric dermatosis

This indicates a group of chronic benign conditions of unknown cause characterized by increased capillary fragility or permeability

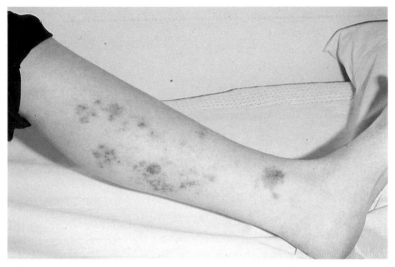

Figure 9.10 **Pigmented purpuric dermatosis.** Asymptomatic brown patches which were localized to the left leg in this boy.

(Figure 9.10). Histopathology reveals a lymphocytic vasculitis with extravasation of red blood cells and haemosiderin deposition. Clinically, dark-red or brown patches of purpura and haemosiderin are seen. The lower legs tend to be the site particularly affected. Usually asymptomatic, more widespread forms with pruritus and lichenification due to persistent scratching are sometimes seen. The prognosis in a particular patient is difficult to forecast but the tendency is to chronicity although some cases do clear within a year.

CHILBLAINS (perniosis)

These are localized inflammatory lesions that arise as an abnormal reaction to cold (Figure 9.11). They are usually seen in homes lacking central heating. They occur especially on fingers, toes, thighs, nose and ears. Affected areas have a cyanotic appearance and can ulcerate. They may occur over local accumulations of fat such as the wrists of infants; at this site the skin may be swollen and feel cold but may be normal in colour. Treatment is warm (but not too tight) clothing and adequate home heating.

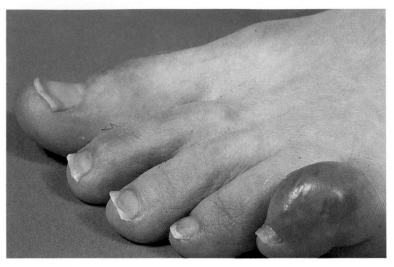

Figure 9.11 **Chilblains.** Florid chilblain of little toe in a 13-year-old girl.

DRUG ERUPTIONS (Figures 9.12–9.15)

Scratch marks

It should be remembered that pruritus may precede a drug eruption and in fact can occur without a rash ever appearing. Severe pruritus will be accompanied by scratching.

Exanthematic drug eruptions

This term indicates a widespread crythematous maculo-papular eruption which may be morbilliform. Ampicillin and phenytoin are common causes. Ampicillin eruptions arc usually exanthematic and appear 5–14 days after starting treatment. Almost all patients with infectious mononucleosis given ampicillin early in the course of infection, develop a distinct irritant copper-coloured purpuric maculo-papular eruption over the trunk and then limbs, 7–10 days after starting antibiotic therapy; the same eruption may occur much less commonly with other penicillins.

Urticaria, erythema multiforme, toxic erythema

Urticaria has been discussed earlier under vascular disorders but drugs are an important cause. Erythema multiforme and toxic erythema have also been mentioned earlier.

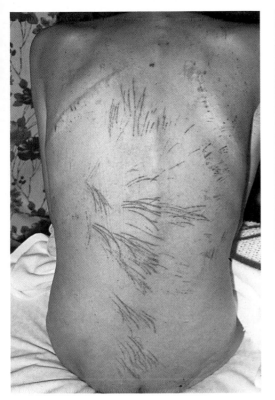

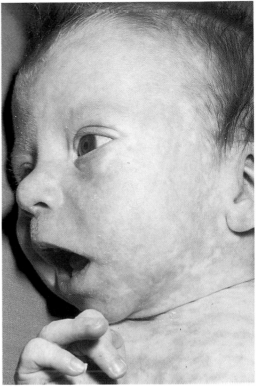

Figure 9.12 **Drug eruption.** Scratch marks in a girl of 15 years with intense itching. This preceded an exanthematic eruption due to a diuretic prescribed in high dosage for cardiac failure.

Figure 9.13 **Drug eruption.** Exanthematic eruption over face in a 2-month-old girl due to amoxycillin.

Corticosteroids

Topical corticosteroids These are most effective external remedies but they are suppressive rather than curative. Short-term use is the aim: The doctor must prevent the patient's skin becoming addicted to the preparation. The more potent ones particularly, can give rise to striae which are usually irreversible and skin atrophy which is often reversible. Both epidermal and dermal atrophy with increased skin fragility, telangiectases, poikilodermatous change and loss of subcutaneous tissue can occur. Even small quantities of a steroid preparation stronger than hydrocortisone cream or hydrocortisone ointment applied to the face for prolonged periods can produce marked skin atrophy and even hydrocortisone itself should not be over-applied to a child's skin. Excessive growth of hair is occasionally seen at the site

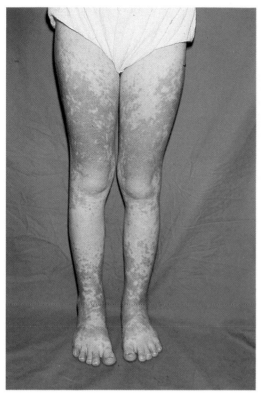

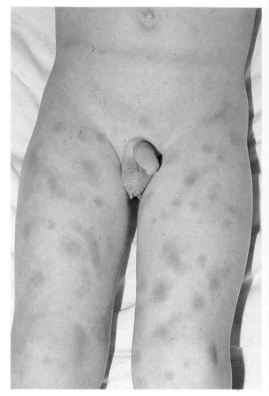

Figure 9.14 **Drug eruption.** Girl of 6 years with florid exanthem which was most marked over limbs. She had received amoxycillin, ampicillin, and erythromycin, and ampicillin was considered the most likely cause.

Figure 9.15 **Drug eruption.** Urticaria attributed to a cough medicine in a 8-year-old boy.

of prolonged steroid application and infection is not an uncommon side-effect in view of the lowered resistance produced by steroid inhibition of the normal inflammatory response. Applications, particularly under occlusion, of potent and usually fluorinated steroids, may lead to interference with pituitary–adrenal function and retard growth. It should be remembered that disposable nappies and particularly plastic pants are occlusive.

Oral corticosteroids These administered on an intermittent basis, on alternate days, will cause less hypothalamic–pituitary–adrenal suppression than daily divided doses.

Local reactions to vaccines

These are included under this section for convenience.

Bacillus Calmette–Guérin vaccine (BCG)   Ulcers and abscesses may follow too deep injection of BCG vaccine (Figure 9.16). Hypertrophic and keloid scars may develop after prolonged site infection. Granulomata, including lupus vulgaris, also occur[4].

Triple vaccine (diphtheria, tetanus, whooping cough)   Persistent nodules may form at the site of injection of triple vaccine particularly adsorbed vaccine. Itching, eczema, hypertrichosis, and hyperpigmentation may occasionally appear at injection sites[5]; such children are often atopic.

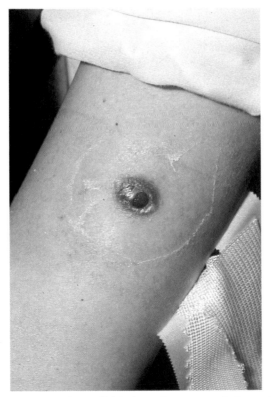

Figure 9.16   **BCG reaction.** Superficial ulceration present 4–5 months after inoculation in a boy of 12 years. No bacterial growth from swab culture. Such ulcers usually heal spontaneously but cleaning with saline may be helpful. Usually the author prescribes 3% chlortetracycline ointment for persistent ulceration.

REFERENCES

1. Warin, R. P. (1987). Urticaria. In Verbov, J. (ed.) *Treatment in Dermatology*, Ch. 4, pp. 93–144. (Lancaster: MTP)
2. Muhlemann, M. F. and Wright, D. J. M. (1987). Emerging pattern of Lyme disease in the United Kingdom and Irish Republic. *Lancet*, **1**, 260-2
3. Imbach, P., Wagner, H. P., Berchtold, W., Gaedicke, G., Hurt, A., Joller, P., Meuller-Eckhardt, C., Muller, B., Rossi, E., and Barandun, S. (1985). Intravenous immunoglobulin versus oral corticosteroids in acute immune thrombocytopenic purpura in childhood. *Lancet*, **2**, 464-8
4. Verbov, J. L. (1984). Local skin complications of BCG vaccination. *Practitioner,* **228**, 1069-71
5. Orlans, D. and Verbov, J. (1982). Skin reactions after triple vaccine. *Practitioner,* **226**, 1295-6

10

Genodermatoses

CONTENTS

AUTOSOMAL DOMINANT

Ichthyosis vulgaris

This is the most common of the many ichthyotic disorders (Figure 10.1). Excessive scaling usually appears during early childhood. The scales are generally small, white and fine, with the flexures characteristically spared. However, over the shins, scales are often large resembling fish-scales. Accentuated palmar and plantar markings are usual.

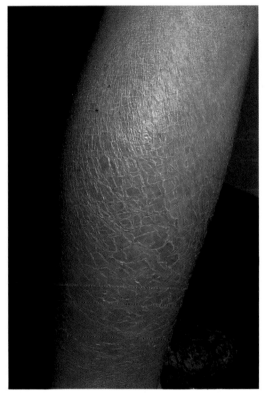

Figure 10.1 **Ichthyosis vulgaris** in a boy of 5½ years.

Tylosis (diffuse palmoplantar keratoderma)

This is the commonest form of inherited localized thickening of skin over palms and soles (Figure 10.2). It manifests in early infancy as well-defined, usually diffuse, smooth regular hyperkeratosis of palms and soles. Fissuring may be a problem in severe cases. A rare association

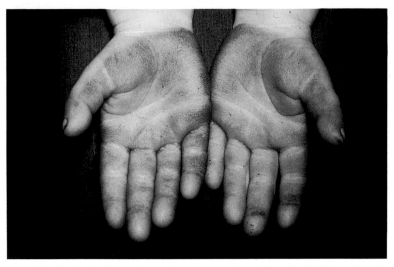

Figure 10.2 **Tylosis.** The change from normal to affected skin is well-defined.

between tylosis appearing in childhood rather than infancy, oral preleukoplakia and/or leukoplakia in tylotic children and adults, and the development of oesophageal carcinoma in adult life, has been described in two Liverpool families.

Ehlers Danlos syndrome (EDS)

This has ten clinically and genetically distinct variants all associated with abnormalities of collagen. Typical features of EDS are hyperextensibility and fragility of the skin with an increased susceptibility to bruising, and hypermobility of the joints (Figure 10.3). The most common types (EDS I, II and III) are inherited in an autosomal dominant manner. The skin has a velvety feel and a fold may be easily stretched returning to its normal position when released. The skin tends to split as a result of relatively minor trauma. Joints are easily dislocated and the condition may present with congenital dislocation of the hip.

Tuberous sclerosis

This is primarily a defect of connective tissue (Figure 10.4). The skin lesions often termed adenoma sebaceum but actually angiofibromata, usually appear towards the end of the first decade as small red-brown papules on the nose and naso-labial folds. They are often mistaken for

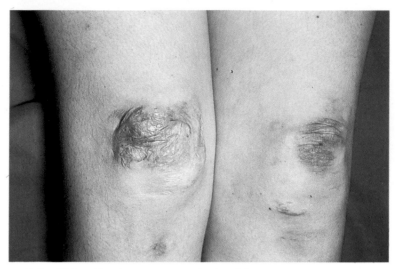

Figure 10.3 **Ehlers–Danlos syndrome.** Ugly diffuse atrophic gaping scars over knees.

acne, which can be distinguished by its more peripheral distribution, the presence of blackheads, and its tendency to form pustules. Other characteristic lesions are fibromas of the nail-folds, irregularly coarsened skin over the sacrum (shagreen patch), and oval hypo-pigmented areas (ash leaf macules), which are usually the earliest skin

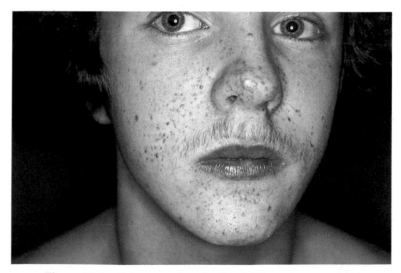

Figure 10.4 **Tuberous sclerosis.** Angiofibromata over face.

sign and often present in the neonate. A smooth red or yellow plaque over the forehead may also be an early sign of the condition[1].

Neurofibromatosis

Multiple benign tumours of neural tissue and multiple café-au-lait patches (six or more of 1.5 cm or more in diameter after puberty are diagnostic) áre usual (Figure 10.5). Although café-au-lait patches usually develop within the first year of life and may be present at birth (see Chapter 2), the cutaneous neurofibromas do not develop until late childhood. Bilateral axillary freckling is pathognomonic of neurofibromatosis. Soft tumours can give the impression of being pushed through a button-hole defect of the skin. Congenital bone anomalies are not uncommon and tumours of brain, spinal cord and peripheral nerves occur.

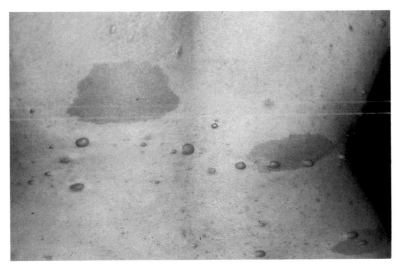

Figure 10.5 **Neurofibromatosis.** Café-au-lait patches and tumours are visible.

Peutz–Jeghers syndrome

In this condition (Figure 10.6) pigmented macules (lentigines) usually appear in infancy or early childhood most commonly in the mouth and on and around the lips but often also over the hands and feet. Polyposis of the small and/or large bowel is part of the syndrome. Although the polyps are usually benign there is a slight but definite increased risk of gastro-intestinal carcinoma. Polyps may also bleed

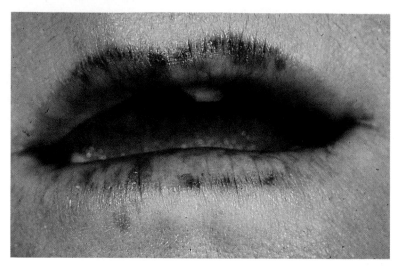

Figure 10.6   **Peutz–Jeghers syndrome** showing characteristic pigmented spots over lips.

leading to anaemia and they also cause intussusception; malaena and abdominal pain may be acute presenting features.

Erythropoietic protoporphyria

This is an uncommon but not rare condition presenting as photo-sensitivity often by the age of 2 years (Figure 10.7). Affected infants are fractious when placed in direct sunlight and older children dislike outdoor activities. Burning or tingling of the face and hands (likened by one of my patients to lemonade fizzing) occur after exposure to sunlight (relevant ultraviolet wavelength is in the 400 nm and longer visible range) and serous crusts may form on the nose; bright windy days are often troublesome. The affected areas develop fine scars. There is an increased incidence of cholelithiasis. Transient fluor-escence of red blood cells confirms the diagnosis. Oral β-carotene is a helpful protective agent in many affected individuals.

Darier's disease (keratosis follicularis)

This is a peculiar dyskeratosis in which distinctive warty, greasy, crusted papules occur over trunk, face, scalp and flexures. White papules may occur on the palate, nail changes including longitudinal white or dark streaks are common, and palms and soles may show

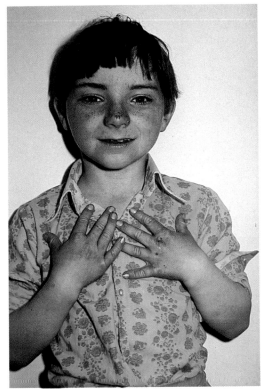

Figure 10.7 **Erythropoietic protoporphyria.** Lesions over nose and knuckles which left characteristic scars.

minute pits interrupting ridges, punctate keratoses and keratoderma. Exacerbations tend to occur in the warmer weather.

Porokeratosis of Mibelli

In this condition lesions are single or multiple and are persistent, usually appearing in childhood and more commonly in males. Lesions are circinate plaques with a raised hyperkeratotic border and sites favoured are face, neck and upper limbs.

AUTOSOMAL RECESSIVE

Acrodermatitis enteropathica

This is seen, particularly in infants at the time of weaning (Figures 10.8–10.10). Exudative eczematous lesions appear around orifices

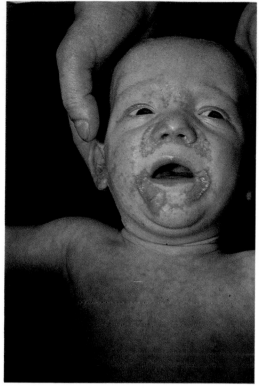

Figure 10.8 **Acrodermatitis enteropathica.** Male of 4 months with typical moist perioral eruption.

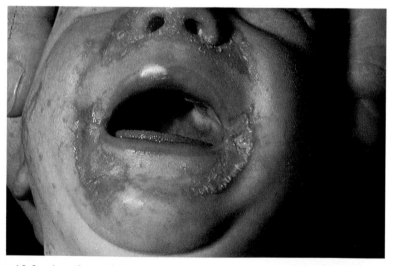

Figure 10.9 **Acrodermatitis enteropathica.** Close-up of same infant as in Figure 10.8.

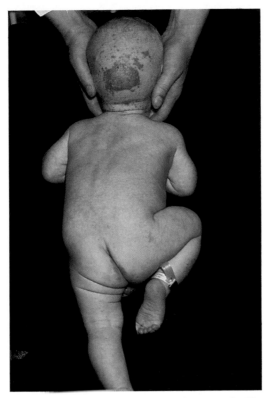

Figure 10.10   **Acrodermatitis enteropathica.** Same infant as in Figures 10.8 and 10.9 showing posterior scalp and natal cleft eruption.

and over scalp, hands and feet. There is diarrhoea, and hair loss from the scalp, eyebrows and eyelashes. This condition is thought to be due to a defect in the absorption of zinc from the bowel and oral zinc sulphate effectively relieves the condition. Zinc deficiency can also be an acquired disorder resulting from inadequate dietary intake, increased zinc loss or intravenous hyperalimentation. Even in the breast-fed infant, whether premature or full-term, low levels of zinc in breast milk may precipitate zinc deficiency[2].

Xeroderma pigmentosum

This is a rare condition characterized by hypersensitivity to ultraviolet rays followed eventually by the development of multiple tumours including solar keratoses, basal and squamous-cell carcinomas and malignant melanomas, in the exposed areas. Photosensitivity may be apparent from the age of 2 months, erythema occurring over exposed areas, particularly the face. After a few years of exposure the skin becomes dry, with freckles, hypopigmentation, atrophy and scarring. Patients may die in childhood from tumour metastases but with modern education, including use of sunscreens, much advice can be given. The cause is a defect of the normal repair mechanism of DNA damaged by ultraviolet rays. The condition can be identified before birth.

X-LINKED RECESSIVE

Chronic granulomatous disease of childhood

This is a disorder affecting boys in the first year of life. Severe recurrent and chronic granulomatous reactions to a number of common bacteria of low virulence occur. There is a defect in the ability of peripheral leucocytes to kill bacteria although cells can phagocytose organisms. This defect is detectable by the inability of patient's cells to reduce the dye nitro-blue tetrazolium. Apart from the skin, lymph nodes, lungs, liver and bone marrow are prone to infection. Long-term antibiotic therapy is important and genetic counselling must be offered.

ECTODERMAL DYSPLASIAS

Focal dermal hypoplasia (Goltz syndrome)

This manifests as scar-like lesions, atrophy and telangiectasia. Over the face the appearance may simulate over-use of the more potent topical corticosteroids. Hypotrichosis, and short partially absent, brittle nails are common. Subcutaneous fat covered only by epidermis may occur over posterior thigh, groin, and iliac crest areas. The X-linked dominant trait is often pre-natally lethal in the male.

Anhidrotic ectodermal dysplasia (Figures 10.11 and 10.12)

This is an X-linked recessive condition in which affected individuals tend to show a similar facial appearance with the nose saddle-shaped with a depressed bridge, the chin small and pointed and the forehead bossed. The skin tends to be pale, soft, thin, dry and shiny. Periorbital skin is wrinkled and hyperpigmented. Scalp hair is short, fine, light

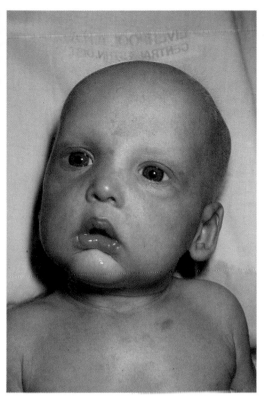

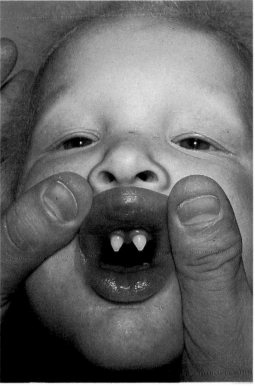

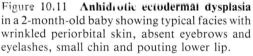

Figure 10.11 **Anhidrotic ectodermal dysplasia** in a 2-month-old baby showing typical facies with wrinkled periorbital skin, absent eyebrows and eyelashes, small chin and pouting lower lip.

Figure 10.12 **Anhidrotic ectodermal dysplasia.** A child aged 3 years showing characteristic pointed 'tiger teeth'. Note absent eyebrows.

in colour, and scanty with eyebrows and eyelashes sparse or absent. Atopic eczema or other manifestations of atopy may be present. There is abnormal, delayed or absent dentition, affecting both the deciduous and permanent teeth. The deciduous teeth are widely spaced and conical. Eccrine sweat glands are absent or diminished in number and total sweating is slight. The nose is often blocked by crusts. Female carriers may show some manifestations such as abnormal dentition, thin scalp hair, reduced sweating and dermatoglyphic abnormalities[3]. It should be noted that in the infant, many characteristic features of the condition are often not apparent and fever of obscure origin may be the only manifestation. It must be emphasized that an infective cause, particularly chest infection should always be looked for in febrile episodes and treated accordingly. Management consists of avoidance of heat and exercise beyond the patient's capacity but affected individuals do tend to show an improved tolerance to environmental heat with age. Dentures will usually be required before school age.

Hypomelanosis of Ito (incontinentia pigmenti achromians)

This presents as widespread asymmetrical and bizarre hypopigmented hypohidrotic areas. Although it appears like a negative image of incontinentia pigmenti, neither verrucous changes nor inflammation precede the depigmentation. Although skin alone may be affected, other abnormalities may be present particularly motor and mental retardation. Skin involvement may appear at, or shortly after, birth but sometimes years later. The cause is generally assumed to be an autosomal dominant gene[4].

Rothmund–Thomson syndrome (poikiloderma congenitale)

This is a rare recessively inherited syndrome, characterized by atrophy, pigmentation and telangiectasia of the skin, in association with juvenile cataracts, short stature, partial or total alopecia, defects of nails and teeth and hypogonadism. It is more common in females. Skin changes generally appear in the first six months of life. There is light-sensitivity with erythema with or without blisters occurring on exposed skin, although the subsequent poikiloderma and other changes are not confined to sites of exposure.

Other genodermatoses are discussed in Chapter 2.

REFERENCES

1. Fryer, A. E., Osborne, J. P. and Schutt, W. (1987). Forehead plaque: a presenting skin sign in tuberous sclerosis. *Arch. Dis. Child.*, **62**, 292–3
2. Roberts, L. J., Shadwick, C. F. and Bergstresser, P. R. (1987). Zinc deficiency in two full-term breast-fed infants. *J. Am. Acad. Dermatol.*, **16**, 301–4
3. Verbov, J. (1970). Hypohidrotic (or anhidrotic) ectodermal dysplasia—an appraisal of diagnostic methods. *Br. J. Dermatol.*, **83**, 341–8
4. Freire-Maia, N. and Pinheiro, M. (1984). *Ectodermal dysplasias: A Clinical and Genetic Study*. Ch. 3, pp. 63–5. (New York: Alan R. Liss Inc.)

11

Non-hereditary Bullous Diseases and Mastocytoses

CONTENTS

NON-HEREDITARY BULLOUS DISEASES

Chronic bullous disease of childhood (linear IgA dermatosis of childhood)

This is the most frequently seen of the three rare conditions in this section (the other two being dermatitis herpetiformis and bullous pemphigoid). It usually begins before the age of six and presents with tense bullae of varying sizes, some haemorrhagic, arising on normal or erythematous skin (Figure 11.1). The lower half of the trunk, genitalia, and lower limbs are most commonly affected sites. Pruritus is variable. Blisters often occur in small ringed patterns. Histopathology reveals a subepidermal bulla with a variable dermal infiltrate. Direct immunofluorescence will usually demonstrate linear IgA deposition along the basement membrane (Figure 11.2). A circulating IgA basement

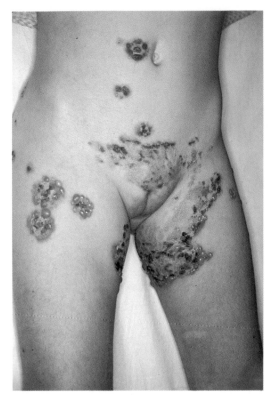

Figure 11.1 **Chronic bullous disease of childhood.** Rosettes of blisters are particularly well-shown over the right thigh (courtesy of Dr. T. W. Stewart).

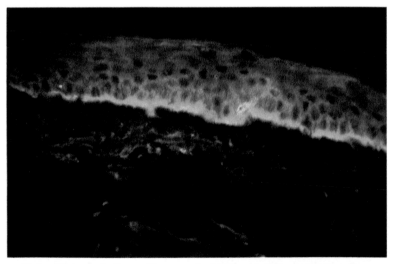

Figure 11.2 **Chronic bullous disease of childhood.** Direct immunofluorescence showing linear deposition of IgA (courtesy of Prof. S. S. Bleehen).

membrane zone antibody is also present in up to 80% of cases. The condition is subject to remissions and may clear spontaneously within 2-3 years. Dapsone (diaminodiphenylsulphone) in as low a dose as 20 mg daily may be helpful but it should be remembered that this a drug with many side-effects including adverse effects on the blood. Conjunctival scarring may occur and regular ophthalmological examination is essential.

Dermatitis herpetiformis

In childhood this is the same pruritic condition as in the adult, but it has an age of onset from 6–11 years. Grouped vesicles and urticated papules occur. Immunofluorescent studies will show a granular IgA deposition at the dermo–epidermal junction, especially in dermal papillae in uninvolved skin. C3 may also be present.

The majority of patients with dermatitis herpetiformis have an enteropathy, demonstrated by jejunal biopsy, identical to that of coeliac disease. Treatment with a gluten-free diet in such patients will produce improvement in both skin and bowel but skin improvement may take many months to be obvious. Dapsone is usually also given initially; if the degree of itching is severe, a dosage of 25–50 mg a day is given. Most cases of dermatitis herpetiformis persist into adult life but periods of remission are common.

Bullous pemphigoid

In children this appears in the under-six age group. Crops of tense bullae, which may be blood-stained, occur on normal or erythematous skin especially over the face, genito-crural regions, and limbs. It is not pruritic. The subepidermal bullae may be accompanied by a mostly eosinophilic dermal infiltrate. Mucous membranes may be affected. Direct immunofluorescence shows linear basement membrane staining for IgG in lesional skin and IgA, IgM and C3 may also be present. Indirect immunofluorescence can be used to demonstrate a circulating IgG antibody against basement membrane. Treatment in children is usually with oral corticosteroids. The condition tends to be self-limiting and usually clears before puberty.

MASTOCYTOSES

These are uncommon conditions in which there are accumulations of mast cells in the skin. Occasionally there may be involvement of other tissues, notably bone.

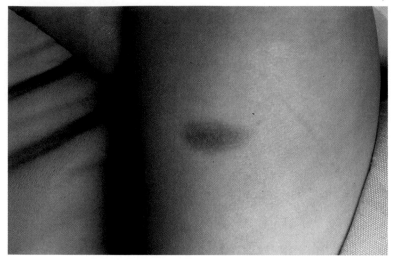

Figure 11.3 **Mast-cell naevus.** This thigh lesion appeared at 2 weeks of age in this 8-month-old child and showed some urtication on rubbing.

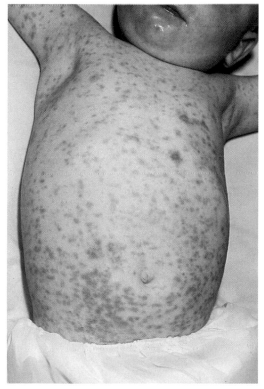

Figure 11.4 **Urticaria pigmentosa.** A 14-month old child with widespread maculo-papular lesions. It began at 2 months.

Mast-cell naevus

This appears as a solitary (Figure 11.3) or a few nodules which may blister at times, in infants and young children.

Diffuse cutaneous mastocytosis

In this rare form characteristic leathery induration of the skin which may take months to develop occurs. This form of mastocytosis is more likely to be associated with internal spread.

Urticaria pigmentosa

This is the most common variety of mast-cell disease. Lesions may be present at birth or appear in the first nine months of life (Figures 11.4 and 11.5). The typical lesion is a small brown-red macule or papule which blanches on pressure and urticates after rubbing. Dermographism is commonly present. Symptoms may be absent or there may be itching or flushing. Long-standing lesions show pigmentation. Oral terfenadine or hydroxyzine may control symptoms but in more severe cases oral sodium cromoglycate which blocks mast-cell degranulation is also useful. The tendency in children is for resolution to occur. In most cases of urticaria pigmentosa, no family history of the condition is obtained but familial cases suggesting autosomal dominant or recessive inheritance have been described.

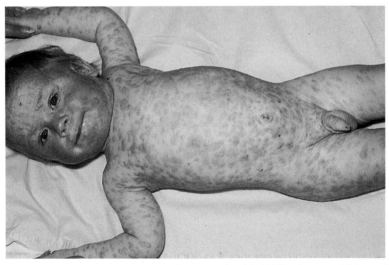

Figure 11.5 **Urticaria pigmentosa.** This 8-month-old child had more widespread and more florid lesions and was subject to flushing attacks due to histamine release.

All the above forms may show vesicular or bullous variants and widespread blistering may mimic staphylococcal scalded skin syndrome or blistering dermatoses. It should be noted that the skin of the infant blisters more easily than in older individuals.

Mastocytosis has been usefully reviewed recently[1].

REFERENCE

1. Stein, D. H. (1986). Mastocytosis: A review. *Pediatr. Dermatol.*, **3**, 365–75

12

Acne, Trauma, Light Eruptions and Pigmentation Disorders

CONTENTS

ACNE

Infantile acne

This appears between the age of 3 and 4 months and 5 years (Figure 12.1). When acne does occur in children under 3 months of age it is sometimes referred to as *acne neonatorum* and it is more common in boys. In the great majority of cases of infantile acne there is no

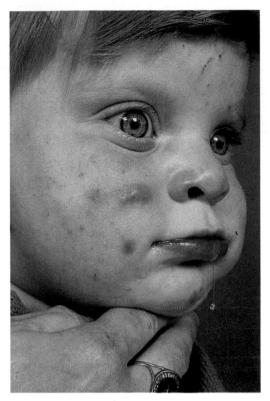

Figure 12.1 **Infantile acne** in 1-year-old boy with florid cheek lesions.

evidence of endocrine disorder. Papules, pustules, nodules and cysts occur and there may be comedones. Most cases improve within a few years but some of these children tend to clear only to develop severe acne at adolescence. Treatment includes topical sulphur (1–3%) in a cream, although in more severe cases benzoyl peroxide preparations may be used. In view of the possibility of yellow or yellow-brown discoloration of deciduous or permanent teeth occurring with oral tetracyclines, these should be avoided not only in pregnancy but also in children up to the age of 12 years. Oral erythromycin can be prescribed in children with severe inflammatory acne.

Acne vulgaris (common acne)

In its mild form (Figure 12.2) this is so common between the ages of 14 and 19 years that it may be considered physiological. However,

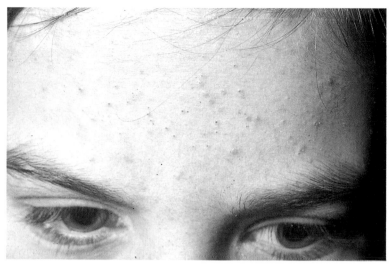

Figure 12.2 **Acne vulgaris.** Blackheads are prominent over the forehead in this 12-year-old.

it can be severe (Figure 12.3) and produce both physical and mental discomfort. Aetiological factors in acne include increased sebum production, comedogenesis, microbial colonization of the pilosebaceous duct and the production of inflammation. Use of ordinary soap and water is to be encouraged. Topical treatments include benzoyl

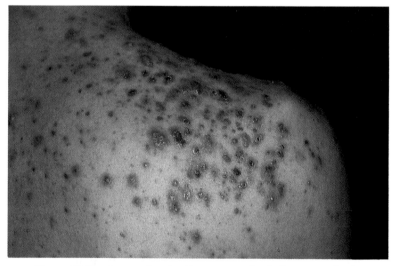

Figure 12.3 **Acne vulgaris.** Severe pustular lesions over back.

peroxide and retinoic acid creams, and oral tetracyclines are the first-line oral antibiotic therapy. It should be noted that adolescents may respond to acne treatment more slowly than older individuals.

TRAUMA

Child abuse

This includes physical and emotional neglect as well as *non-accidental injury* (NAI), a term that includes sexual abuse. NAI (Figure 12.4) may be visible in the skin as bruising, abrasions, burns, ulceration or hair loss and it is essential practice to notice any signs of trauma when fully examining a child's skin.

Sexual abuse may present with allegations by the child or an adult, injuries to genitalia or anus or suspicious features such as unexplained recurrent urinary infections. Although there is little doubt that sexual

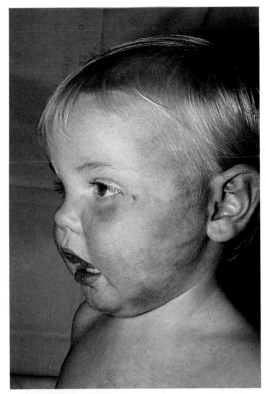

Figure 12.4 **Non-accidental injury.** Bruising and swelling over face.

abuse has been under-diagnosed in the past, it is a diagnosis that should be made with great care. It should be appreciated that masturbation is common in children of all ages, that children bathe together or with parents or share the parents' bed and this does not constitute sexual abuse.

If there is good reason to suspect NAI, the child should be undressed completely and examined fully with a nurse and preferably parent also present, and relevant findings documented with drawings. If suspicions are not allayed the child should be admitted under the care of a Consultant Paediatrician experienced in child abuse. If the parents refuse to agree to the child being admitted, a Place of Safety Order may be sought which allows the child to be kept in hospital for up to 28 days. A rapid coordinated approach by doctors, social workers, health visitors, people who know the family and the police, is necessary to plan investigations in cases of NAI.

Black heel syndrome (talon noir)

This syndrome is a common asymptomatic condition occurring in athletic adolescents, particularly football and basketball players. Clusters of black specks appear at the back or side of the heel just above the hyperkeratotic edge of the foot (Figures 12.5 and 12.6). Lesions resemble a tattoo and may be mistaken for plantar warts or even malignant melanoma. However, black heel tends to be bilateral

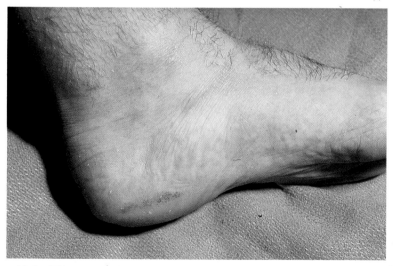

Figure 12.5 **Black heel.** Linear black spots over inner heel. Note the localization to a frictional site.

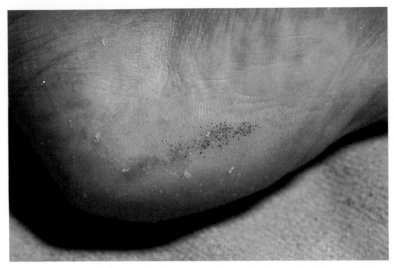

Figure 12.6 **Black heel.** Close-up of same lesion as in Figure 12.5

and symmetrical. It is usually noted early in the playing season and hardness of the ground seems relevant. Papillary capillaries are ruptured by the shearing action associated with the sport.

Dermatitis artefacta

A child presents, usually an older girl, in whom deliberate self-mutilation of the skin is suspected (Figure 12.7). The resulting ulceration, excoriation, or purpura is bizarre in appearance and invariably accessible to self-infliction. Characteristically, occluded lesions heal rapidly only to recur with further exposure. It usually occurs in intellectually dull and unsophisticated children as a form of attention-seeking or protest. Usually a histrionic gesture, most cases have no significance beyond a limited nuisance value. Management includes listening carefully to the history of the appearance of the lesions and although you may take a parent into your confidence in some instances, usually you should not directly accuse the patient of deliberately producing lesions; she will not attend for follow-up if you do. Rarely, early schizophrenia may present in this way in the adolescent.

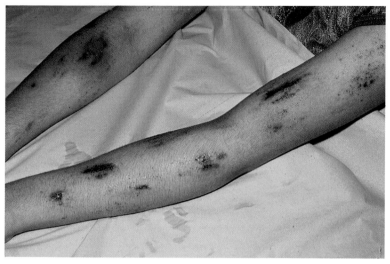

Figure 12.7 **Dermatitis artefacta.** Scratched excoriated arm lesions. She also had similar facial lesions and had seen other consultants of various disciplines with recurrent bruising inferior to the right eye, also self-inflicted in fact.

LIGHT ERUPTIONS

Sunburn

This indicates a cutaneous erythema of sufficient degree to cause discomfort (Figure 12.8), caused by sun exposure at wavelengths between 290 and 320 nm (UVB range). Skin signs may vary from a mild erythema to a severe reaction with blister formation. Constitutional symptoms may be severe with extensive sunburn and include nausea, malaise, fever and delirium.

Prophylactic measures are most important and this is particularly essential for infants and fair-skinned children who cannot tolerate sun exposure. Use of hats and long-sleeved clothing in addition to sunscreens with a sun-protection factor (SPF) of at least 8 for such children are important and youngsters not used to regular sunlight exposure must not be exposed for too long a period, particularly during the peak ultraviolet exposure time between 10 a.m. and 2 p.m. Treatment of sunburn includes calamine lotion and mildly potent topical steroids are also useful in severe acute cases.

It is worth noting that childhood sun exposure may be of critical importance in the aetiology of malignant melanoma in adulthood.

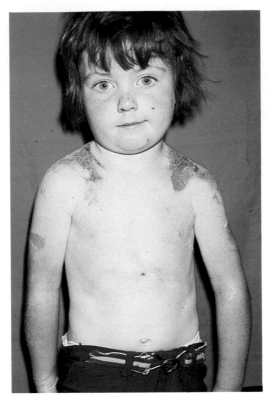

Figure 12.8 **Sunburn.** Boy of 4 years exposed to the sun for too long. An older sibling looking after him forgot about him. His back was more severely burnt.

Polymorphic light eruption

This may start in early childhood but usually first appears in early adult life. It is sometimes familial and is more common in females. Multiple small itchy red papules which may become confluent occur on exposed areas in the summer season. In many patients there is a delay of several hours to a few days between sun exposure and the onset of the eruption. There is a tendency for the eruption to be less severe as the summer progresses in particular patients. Short-wavelength ultraviolet light (290–320 nm) is always involved, but longer wavelengths may also be relevant in some patients.

Actinic prurigo

This is a similar light eruption in which both UVA and UVB may contribute. It is more common in females, and with an onset in childhood. Persistent irritant papules occur not only on exposed sites but often

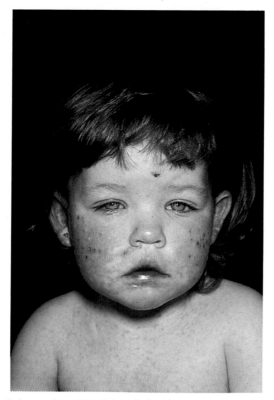

Figure 12.9 **Actinic prurigo.** Tearful and showing excoriated papules over cheeks.

also on covered areas such as sacrum and buttocks. Flat scars may occur over the face and forehead. The papules are often excoriated showing weeping and crusting (Figure 12.9). In some cases it may be present all the year round but with worsening in summer. Prognosis is variable but many children clear after a period of years. Management includes advice on suitable clothing, restriction of UV exposure, and use of sun-screening agents with a high SPF.

Erythropoietic protoporphyria, xeroderma pigmentosum and *Rothmund–Thomson syndrome* have been mentioned in Chapter 10.

PIGMENTATION DISORDERS

Oculocutaneous albinism

This results from failure of melanocytes in skin, hair and eye to synthesize normal amounts of melanin (Figure 12.10). The condition is inherited as an autosomal recessive trait. The skin colour is light and

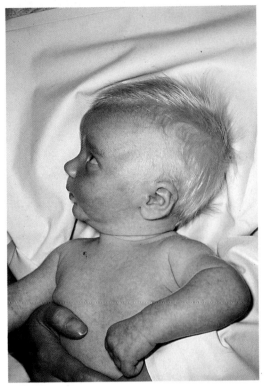

Figure 12.10 **Oculocutaneous albinism.** Note the silvery-white hair in this infant who had tyrosinase-positive albinism. His hair will tend to darken with age and he may also show some ability to tan.

the hair whitish-yellow. The skin is very sensitive to solar radiation with the common appearance in time of solar keratoses and skin carcinoma. There is also photophobia, reduced visual acuity and nystagmus. The two most common types of oculocutaneous albinism are the tyrosinase-negative and tyrosinase-positive types. In the negative type, hair incubated *in vitro* with tyrosine and DOPA will fail to darken but in the positive type, hair bulbs darken readily. From a clinical point of view, some pigment is formed in the positive type and they may have the ability to tan. In addition their visual acuity may improve as they get older. Restriction of UV exposure and use of a high SPF sun-screen are, of course, essential.

Vitiligo

This is a common distressing disorder said to occur in 1% of the world population (Figures 12.11–12.13). In about half of the affected

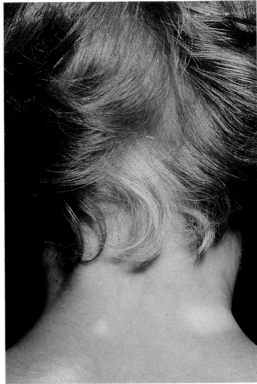

Figure 12.11 **Vitiligo.** Widespread over trunk.

Figure 12.12 **Vitiligo.** Same boy as in Figure 12.11 with white hair visible over posterior scalp.

individuals it develops before the age of 20 years. The aetiology is unknown but between 30–40% of patients have a positive family history. There is a marked absence of melanocytes and melanin in the affected epidermis. Although usually symmetrical, vitiligo may be unilateral, and a dermatomal (segmental) arrangement is seen more commonly in children than in adults[1]. Management of the condition is unsatisfactory but cosmetic cover sometimes and use of sun-screen applications are indicated.

Erythema dyschromicum perstans (ashy dermatosis)

This was first described in 1957 in El Salvador. Most cases have come from Central, North and South America. It is a chronic disease of unknown aetiology, but without systemic effects. Of equal sex incidence it usually presents in early adult life, but children over the

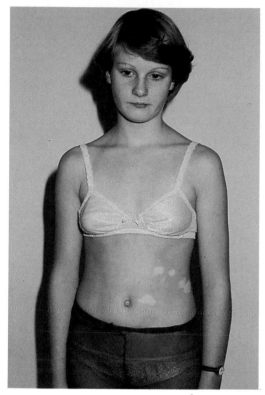

Figure 12.13 **Vitiligo.** This girl of 14 years shows unilateral localized segmental vitiligo.

age of 5 years can be affected. Widespread asymptomatic or slightly irritant slate-grey macules or plaques appear over trunk and limbs and active lesions may show a raised edge. Although chronic, the condition does tend to resolve.

Kwashiorkor

This is seen in starving children and is characterized by localized or generalized oedema, apathy, anorexia, growth retardation, diarrhoea and skin changes (Figure 12.14). The condition mostly affects children from 4 months to 4 years of age and the most striking skin manifestation is hyperpigmented scaly plaques especially prominent on the limbs. They peel leaving hypopigmented macules. Chronic pellagra lesions in contrast are localized to light-exposed areas. Apart from the plaques, the skin is generally dry and atrophic. Diffuse hair loss,

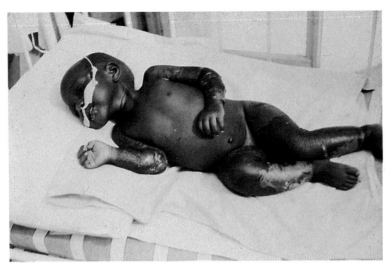

Figure 12.14 **Kwashiorkor** in an 18-month-old infant from The Gambia showing hyperpigmented plaques over limbs and some hypopigmented areas (courtesy of Prof. R. G. Hendrickse).

haemorrhagic blisters, large areas of erosion, and secondary bacterial infection also occur. Treatment of the dry skin is with emollients and infection should also be treated. However, correction of the underlying malnutrition is the main priority in treatment. It should be remembered that kwashiorkor can also occur in malnourished children in an affluent society.

REFERENCE

1. Halder, R. M., Grimes, P. E., Cowan, C. A., Enterline, J. A., Chakrabarti, S. G. and Kenney, Jr, J. A. (1987). Childhood vitiligo. *J. Am. Acad. Dermatol.*, **16**, 948–54

Appendix 1: A Selection of Recommended Prescribable Proprietary Topical and Oral Preparations

EMOLLIENTS

- Alcoderm (liquid paraffin in moisturizing base)
- Aquadrate (urea 10%)
- Diprobase cream (liquid paraffin, white soft paraffin, ceto-macrogol, cetostearyl alcohol)
- Diprobase ointment (liquid paraffin, white soft paraffin)
- Eczederm (calamine, arachis oil)
- Neutrogena Norwegian Formula Hand Cream (includes glycerin, cetearyl alcohol, cetearyl sulphate) – over the counter *only*
- Nutraplus (urea 10%)
- Ultrabase (white soft paraffin, liquid paraffin, stearyl alcohol)
- Unguentum (silicic acid, liquid paraffin, white soft paraffin, polysorbate-40, glycerol monostearate, saturated neutral oil, sorbic acid, propylene glycol)

Bath emollients

- Alpha Keri (liquid paraffin, lanolin oil)
- Aveeno oilated (colloidal oat, liquid paraffin)
- Balneum (soya oil)
- Emulsiderm (liquid paraffin, isopropyl myristate, benzalkonium chloride)
- Hydromol (light liquid paraffin, isopropyl myristate)
- Oilatum (liquid paraffin, acetylated wool alcohols)

TOPICAL STEROIDS (as creams or ointments and with or without other constituents)

Mildly potent

- Efcortelan and many others (hydrocortisone base or acetate)— Some of the other preparations of hydrocortisone are now available without a prescription over the counter.
- Modrasone (alclometasone dipropionate)
- Nystaform-HC (hydrocortisone, chlorhexidine, nystatin)
- Synalar 1:10 (fluocinolone acetonide)
- Terra-Cortril (hydrocortisone, oxytetracycline hydrochloride)
- Vioform-hydrocortisone (hydrocortisone, clioquinol)

Moderately potent

- Alphaderm (hydrocortisone, urea)
- Calmurid HC (hydrocortisone, urea, lactic acid)
- Haelan (flurandrenolone)
- Haelan C (flurandrenolone, clioquinol)
- Trimovate (clobetasone butyrate, nystatin, oxytetracycline (in cream) or chlortetracycline (in ointment))
- Ultradil (fluocortolone pivalate, fluocortolone hexanoate)

Potent

- Betnovate-RD (betamethasone valerate)
- Locoid-C (hydrocortisone 17-butyrate, chlorquinaldol)
- Propaderm-A (beclomethasone dipropionate, chlortetracycline hydrochloride)

SCABIES

- Ascabiol (benzyl benzoate 25%)
- Derbac-M, Prioderm (malathion 0.5%)
- Eurax (crotamiton 10%)
- Lorexane, Quellada (lindane 1%)

HEAD LICE

- Derbac shampoo (carbaryl 0.5%)
- Derbac-M, Prioderm, Suleo-M (malathion 0.5%)
- Esoderm (lindane 1%)

WARTS—particularly for plantar warts

- Cuplex (salicylic acid, lactic acid, copper acetate)
- Glutarol (glutaraldehyde)
- Salactol, Duofilm (salicylic acid, lactic acid)

PSORIASIS

- Alphosyl (coal tar extract, allantoin)
- Carbo-Dome (coal tar solution)
- Clinitar (coal tar extract)
- Dithrocream (dithranol)
- Genisol, Polytar, T-gel are tar shampoos
- Polytar emollient—added to bath

ACNE

- Benoxyl ⎫
- Benzagel ⎬ benzoyl peroxide-containing preparations
- Nericur ⎭

ANTIBACTERIALS

- Achromycin (tetracycline hydrochloride)
- Bactroban (mupirocin)
- Betadine (povidone-iodine)
- Fucidin (fusidic acid)

ANTIFUNGALS

- Exelderm (sulconazole)
- Nizoral (ketoconazole)
- Nystan (nystatin)

ANTIVIRAL

- Zovirax (acyclovir)—Topical, oral and intravenous preparations.

COSMETIC COVER CREAMS include

- Covermark
- Veil

SUN-SCREENS include

- Coppertone Supershade 15 and Ultrashade 23
- Piz Buin cream Nos. 6, 8, 12 and lipstick
- Roc Total sunblock 15 A + B
- Spectraban 4 and 15

ORAL PREPARATIONS

COW'S MILK SUBSTITUTES

- Formula S
- Isomil
- Prosobee
- Wysoy

} All nutritionally complete soya-based milks

- Nutramigen
- Pregestimil

} For children who do not tolerate soya milk these are nutritionally complete preparations containing hydrolyzed protein

ANTIHISTAMINES

- Atarax (hydroxyzine)
- Piriton (chlorpheniramine)
- Tavegil (clemastine)
- Triludan (terfenadine)
- Vallergan (trimeprazine)

Many of the above are available world-wide, often under different trade names. These include some emollients, hydrocortisone and alclometasone, dithranol (known as anthralin), benzoyl peroxide, Nizoral (ketoconazole), Zovirax (acyclovir) and trimeprazine in the USA and Quellada, Alphosyl, Polytar and both urea and benzoyl peroxide-containing preparations in Australia.

Appendix 2: Useful Reading

Journals

- *Pediatric Dermatology* **(all issues)**
  Edited by L. M. Solomon & N. B. Esterly
  Blackwell Scientific Publications, Boston

- *Seminars in Dermatology* **(issue** on *Advances in Pediatric Dermatology,* 1988)
  Edited by J. L. Verbov
  Grune & Stratton Inc., Florida

Books

- *Modern Topics in Paediatric Dermatology,* 1979
  Edited by J. L. Verbov
  Heinemann Medical Books, London

- *Clinical Pediatric Dermatology,* 1981
  S. Hurwitz
  W. B. Saunders Co., Philadelphia

- *Colour Atlas of Paediatric Dermatology,* 1983
  J. Verbov & N. Morley
  MTP, Lancaster

- *The Skin and Systemic Disease in Children,* 1985
  S. Hurwitz
  Year Book Medical Publishers Inc., Chicago

- *Handbook of Pediatric Dermatology,* 1985
  J. I. Harper
  Butterworths, London

- *Practical Pediatric Dermatology*, 2nd Edn., 1985
  W. L. Weston
  Little, Brown & Co., Boston

- *Pediatric Dermatology. Dermatologic Clinics*, January, 1986
  Edited by S. Hurwitz
  W. B. Saunders Co., Philadelphia

- *Atlas of Paediatric Dermatology*, 1986
  C. L. Meneghini & E. Bonifazi
  Martin Dunitz, London

- *Genodermatoses. Dermatologic Clinics*, January, 1987
  Edited by J. C. Alper
  W. B. Saunders Co., Philadelphia

- *Pediatric Dermatology*, 1987
  Edited by R. Happle & E. Grosshans
  Springer-Verlag, Berlin & Heidelberg

- *Vascular Birthmarks*, 1987
  Edited by T. J. Ryan & G. W. Cherry
  Oxford University Press, Oxford

Index